# Live in the Moment

## Change Your Mind and Things Will Change

*(How to Live in the Moment and Live a Stress-free Life Style)*

**Matthew Wurster**

Published By **Tyson Maxwell**

**Matthew Wurster**

*Live in the Moment: Change Your Mind and Things Will Change (How to Live in the Moment and Live a Stress-free Life Style)*

**ISBN   978-1-998038-97-8**

No part of this guidebook shall be reproduced in any form without permission in writing from the publisher except in the case of brief quotations embodied in critical articles or reviews.

Legal & Disclaimer

The information contained in this book is not designed to replace or take the place of any form of medicine or professional medical advice. The information in this book has been provided for educational & entertainment purposes only.

The information contained in this book has been compiled from sources deemed reliable, and it is accurate to the best of the Author's knowledge; however, the Author cannot guarantee its accuracy and validity and cannot be held liable for any errors or omissions. Changes are periodically made to this book. You must consult your doctor or get professional medical advice before using any of the suggested remedies, techniques, or information in this book.

Table Of Contents

## Chapter 1: Accepting The Present And Appreciating It

In the start of the story the farmer wished for a lavish lifestyles. That become some component he turn out to be operating for in his future, however did he respect what he had now?

Did he thank God for what he emerge as provided with nowadays? His youngsters had been healthful; he himself turn out to be healthy as turned into his accomplice. She cherished him, relied on him and helped him. The secure haven! Which such a number of human beings don't have, he had it.

This is what we neglect. We are quick to factor out matters we don't have, but why are we able to neglect about about to apprehend all that we have now?

We want to start appreciating what we've got and do our terrific to get what we don't have. But don't be disenchanted with anything; begin finding the high-quality within the normal!

"I used to win such loads of quizzes all over again then! Now I barely take into account stuff!"

Dwelling on our past accomplishments is some other difficulty we need to do lessen. Now, as you study this you might be wondering: 'but how can I forget about the achievements I've made!'

No one is telling us to surely erase them from our reminiscences. We need not ponder upon them or preserve bringing them up in topics. Like the times pass by way of way of we increase up. We are becoming older and there are changes taking location in our body. Accept them.

At gift, some of us can't consider stuff the manner we did in advance than and there can be no trouble with that. Sometimes, we surely don't bear in mind topics that nicely, however that does not propose that it's the prevent.

We have opportunity solutions.

"I used to stroll miles in advance. But after this coincidence, I can barely walk. What did I do to deserve this?"

It is hard to simply accept some drastic adjustments. But have a look at it in reality. That individual can although stroll! So, in choice to concentrating at the horrific, bear in mind the best.

"Saying all this is simple, but going thru it? You don't recognize the ache!"

We'll come to be realistic the day we start accepting topics the way they're.

We genuinely don't recognise who is going through ache and who isn't. Everyone faces their very very own issues and for absolutely everyone their trouble is equally tough. No one's hassle or ache is extra or lesser.

One concept for this form of scenario is Sean Swarner. He is the primary most cancers survivor to complete the 7 summits, the exceptional peaks of seven international places. The medical doctors gave up on him, they informed him he had 2 weeks to stay. But have a look at the achievements he made after he acquired his warfare with most cancers.

Get up over again and reap what you can from your state now.

Everyday be satisfied approximately all that you have. The garments you're wearing the house you're living in and the food you consume. Be grateful which you are healthful and able to see via the day.

ATTITUDE

Now once I communicate approximately attitude; I am summing it up for, our thoughts-set towards life, the human beings spherical us and ourselves.

Yes, ourselves! How masses can we recognize our choices? How a bargain can we recognize our frame? How an lousy lot can we definitely recognize ourselves?

We want to understand our frame, irrespective of what. Whether we're fats, skinny, have stretch marks, tall or small. It does not rely! You are you and no person can exchange that.

If you begin wondering you aren't as lovable due to the fact the others or are too fat to flaunt that get dressed, then you'll enchantment to all of the ones terrible energies. It will then have an impact on you and start affecting your dating with the others.

How may additionally all of this turn out to be a hassle among my relationships with others?

When you start criticizing yourselves, your mind builds up that photo for your head and in due time you start making conclusions which aren't proper.

You start thinking that perhaps you are like this so, no one will need to satisfy you.That effects in you cancelling your plans. Or, if a person takes an interest in you or wants to start a friendship, you are not assured and emerge as making a fuss in amongst conversations. You experience like locking your self up and end up blaming your self.

So now, when you stand inside the front of the replicate, flex your muscle mass! You are sturdy. You are cute, you are good-looking and no person can take you down. You private yourself and no character can actually will let you understand what you're. You are what you're making of your self.

You are the driving force of your personal life, caretaker of your very non-public body, mind and soul.

You are stunning, sturdy and confident.

Don't blame your internal soul and voice that lets in you in each desire. Don't blame it in case you pass wrong someplace, because of the fact you're in reality blaming your self.

Always anticipate on the brighter facet. At least you have been assured and succesful enough of taking your very personal choice and jogging on it.

You are doing super. Become one collectively with your real self and don't hesitate to just accept the real you.

"The real problem is to conquer the manner you do not forget your self"

Maya Angelou.

Be pleased with your self.

Learning from our errors and doing better or being cautious the subsequent time is what we should do in area of blaming ourselves. Just take delivery of if you have achieved a few aspect incorrect and get beyond it, don't maintain blaming your self for it.

Now, how is our mind-set in the direction of humans round us? How is our thoughts-set in the direction of the ones near us?

Sometimes even as strolling down the street we come upon a person, we speedy express regret.

When we encounter our siblings, are we able to express regret? Instead we blurt out 'Can't you notice?' and stroll away.

We will discover modifications in our thoughts-set within the direction of latest human beings we meet and people we recognize due to the reality we will be predisposed to be greater of our proper selves within the the front of the humans we realize and try to make a extraordinary have an effect on on the ones we don't.

But we want to trade this dependancy a piece.

Why? Because we appear to damage our close to ones and don't even recognise it.

Maybe our sibling had a lousy day already and needs a hug? The least that may be completed is not get angry and stroll away.

We generally have a propensity to pour our anger out on those we recognize, questioning they recognize us and received't select us in any respect.

On the other side we additionally want to remember, what if they'll be going through a hard time and need a few region or hobby?

We do not recognize our parents as tons as we need to. When we had been little, it have become a tremendous hassle. But now that we have got have been given a higher knowledge, we want to begin complimenting them for what they do. If you've got were given a spouse, appreciate their love for you. They care approximately you the equal manner you do for them.

There have become a poem in excessive college in which the poet defined how the mom become truly frustrated from work and at the manner domestic she bumped into her neighbour, to whom she apologized with a smile. When she had been given home and turned into busy making equipped dinner her little daughter ran into her and a few component fell from her hand. This, the mom did no longer be aware of, due to the fact, she fumed in anger and knowledgeable her to get lower again to her room and now not disturb her.

Later she found the lovely flowers tied collectively mendacity near the refrigerator. She picked them up and headed to her daughter's mattress room.

She kissed her brow and apologized. Then her daughter explained how she had determined the flora in the lawn and amassed them to make a lovable small bouquet to surprise her with for her birthday. She end up fame quietly behind her to wonder her. But it all have grow to be out to be different.

 The mother later realised how she had hurt her very own even as she turned into so thoughtful.

And as for the farmer's case, if he might have been careful enough to no longer allow his anger and inflammation display inside the front of his children, who've been too naïve to apprehend matters but, or perhaps lead them to recognize how the scenario become affecting him, they may have shared a higher bond.

So, subsequent time while you feel low, attempt to talk approximately it collectively along side your friends or close to ones in location of maintaining it internal. Otherwise, you'll quick pour out the anger on a person . If you do now not recollect every person, speak for your private thoughts and calm it down.

Try and make a addiction of wishing your own family people 'Good morning, afternoon, nighttime and night time time'. Whenever they'll be heading out, choice them success.

 When they get domestic, ask them how their day turn out to be. It makes a distinction. Just some phrases can make loads of difference.

People these days get indignant over small subjects and end up preventing with their neighbours or surely all of us at the streets.

## Chapter 2: How Can We Try To Save You This?

The trade you carry in yourself will assist you with this. If someone bumps into you and they seem off, express regret and ask, 'are you doing fantastic?'

It is not as masses as us to determine in advance whether or not or no longer the individual will respond or now not. If they don't, don't be too judgmental. It's genuinely as masses as them. It is their desire.

Like it's yours to be kind sufficient to care and ask and not begin lashing with awful mouthed phrases.

What inside the occasion that they do not respond and in fact begin taking walks away. It is their desire to achieve this. Just be the way you are. Trust me, it will all come lower lower back. You receives to satisfy exceptional human beings! Think about that, whisk the glare off your shoulder and stroll proud.

"The international we've got created is a fabricated from our thinking; it can't be modified without converting our own questioning."

Albert Einstein

## APPRECIATE, SMILE AND RESPECT EVERYONE

'I recognize about it. I have a have a have a look at it each day. I cannot apprehend it every day.' This is how maximum people expect.

Even the farmer did not understand his wife's loyalty in the path of him. Did he even recognize how stressful she end up? How his kids expert what he did and furnished them with?

Remember as fast because the receive as real with is damaged it's too tough to supply it decrease returned.

The farmer modified into not even grateful that the human beings of his village extinguished the hearth. If they might have now not finished that, his plant life or maybe his residence could have been a part of the fireside. Only if he cared enough to mingle with human beings or make small communicate or as a minimum been attentive, topics might have been unique.

 He might have diagnosed how tough it end up for human beings to adventure far away for cremation. He have emerge as no longer residing in his present. He become misplaced in his goals of the future.

For no reason, apprehend the person who sources newspaper early morning, the individual that guarantees your courier and meals. They are similar to you, people with emotions and feelings.

The put up man in fee of my area, he is elder to me. The day I obtained my passport he grow to be the simplest to supply the happiness. Receiving my first pen friend letter turned into exciting; he have become the most effective to deliver it to me carefully and on time. So, I do not hesitate to thank him and provide him a tumbler of water.

Once, a shipping man modified into thirsty and he have come to be refused a pitcher of water at someone's house, so he did now not dare to ask me. But as soon as I presented him one, he have come to be pleased.

How can someone deny a glass of water? We need to appearance after every exquisite. It isn't spadework, strive it.

Not virtually them, greet your neighbours even as you spot them. Have a smiling face. Help the ones in need. Like I said in advance, don't hesitate to ask a person if they'll be doing first-class after they seem off.

What is going spherical comes round. Everyone can pay for their deeds in their present existence. There isn't any want to be unhappy if someone is impolite or does not smile again, at least you probable did what you felt like and it'll make you feel higher.

You will surround your self with positivity. You will start feeling properly from the interior, within the coming days you will deal with your troubles better, they obtained't be able to have an impact on you that lousy. You gets thru it all in a few unspecified time in the future. So why consider it and surround your self with terrible emotions?

"Smile. Why? Because, it makes you appealing. It adjustments your temper. It relives strain. And it permits you live excessive best.

Again, thank lord for having first-rate people spherical you. For supplying you with this life and offering you with subjects you have got.

## YESTERDAY'S SOLUTIONS ARE NOT TODAY'S SOLUTIONS

Being too laidback comes with its cons.

Cremation= horrible energy, that is what the farmer idea as quickly as he noticed humans gathering for the cremation rite. What we did no longer see is that, his worry and his horrible mindset from the start towards the scenario created extra negativity; making him irritated and indignant.

He commenced to hate the people of his personal village, no matter the fact that he and his family had been further part of it.

This ended in his kids getting a similar concept within the course of life. His spouse too, finally, began thinking that the hearth have come to be because of terrible spirits.

This is what negativity does to us. Our terrible thoughts trap more useless mind.

Our elders normally don't say subjects for the sake of it. We want to surround

18

ourselves with remarkable energy! That is the reality and we need to paintings on it!

What if the farmer and his own family had more of a awesome outlook in the route of life?

The fireside would've commenced due to the modern climate and lifeless leaves? Maybe the character in charge of searching after the hearth did no longer whole his duty definitely. But blaming the spirits to begin a fireplace? Really??

Not notable the farmer's own family, however different people commenced maintaining apart them too! They stopped looking for vegetable from him or paying them a visit. Did the awful energy are living in his veggies? I might now not be amazed if a person went around announcing that they fell ill because they ate food cooked from the vegetables they furnished from him.

We can't genuinely alternate human beings and what they anticipate, however we're the author of our future and ourselves.

The farmer's wife changed into more of a person dwelling the movement, she become aware about the topics taking area around them. She did now not have a horrible idea; as an possibility she surely cared for the hardships the others were going through.

But we cannot truely blame an individual. It all begins offevolved offevolved with the power. We lure greater negativity even as we recall some element loads and in the long run fall into the lure.

Similar matters may be noticed in our lives. Like wondering how we used to remedy certain subjects decrease lower back then. Well today, such mind gained't assist circulate a rock. The subjects we should buy for Rs.10 back then, we received't even get a lollipop for that fee within the cities!

The international has superior. We want to change consequently or we can be left within the decrease again of.

Never be afraid to analyze. Whether it's coming from a person extra younger or older to you, doesn't rely variety. Accept matters if they will be proper. Do now not allow your ego are to be had amongst.

My parents never hesitate to ask me doubts regarding the usage of the modern generation or new pointers or how topics paintings, and I am in no manner tired of assisting them out or mastering what they want to share.

Rely on God.

We all take delivery of as authentic with in God and agree with in him but it's not precise to rely on him really. The God resides internal us. Visiting temples and holy grounds is non violent and clean.

The farmer did no longer thank God for what he end up furnished with already. But he did not fail to take into account God and blame him when he emerge as in trouble. He depended on God a touch too much.

He have become dissatisfied in God at the same time as he were given decrease decrease again; he idea God did not answer his prayers!

Giving him a 2nd threat was God's way of acknowledging his and his circle of relatives's prayers.

God publications us, he does no longer serve us.

Like referred to in advance, we are the drivers of our private existence. So, God is genuinely supporting us navigate thru it.

In in recent times's global, we slightly have the time to speak with our loved ones. Teaching the younger ones is why we carry out a few rituals. Why are we able to accept as true with in God is out of context.

But we want to take day out and feature that talk. A teenager's thoughts is complete of questions and that they need answers. Otherwise their faith in lifestyles diminishes. They truly received't recognize the properly well worth of factors.

We honestly lead them to sit down despite the truth that for the duration of prayers and get indignant if they don't. They emerge as impatient and that is why they are trying to transport spherical or discover a few aspect to pass their time with. Some hardly ever awareness on the mythological reminiscences narrated in between.

But what if you defined to the kid the essence of performing some element, like praying to God? And why ought to one take a seat down though and pay attention to the prayers. It's the terrific feasible meditation. It clears your mind and strengthens your inner self. It's a manner to get toward God and apprehend his creation, i.E. Us!

Once they get a keep close of factors, they'll be greater trustworthy than you. They always were.

Most of the instances, we ourselves are not aware about why we do amazing subjects.

I'll supply an example. My uncle might constantly shout at me after I cut my nails at night time, despite the fact that I were given damage and it became a necessity. I requested him, why no longer reduce nails at night time time. He emerge as silent for a second and then answered that it brings awful omen. I have become surprised. How can God get angry if I reduce my nail at night time? He became a company believer of this and he informed me that his ancestors used to tell him this.

He became not incorrect approximately their ancestors telling them no longer to lessen nails at night time time, but the factor approximately it being a lousy omen is. Maybe some the ancestors did tell that and it's been passed on. But there's a reason for it.

We have strength. We have mild. It's a boon. Our ancestors lived with lamps and candles. They did no longer have this costly. So performing some element at night emerge as tough for them. Hence, they could restrain themselves from lowering their nails as to not emerge as hurting themselves. Now at the same time as we've mild everywhere and we are able to see honestly. So, there may be no want to restrain ourselves from it. But over the years, humans add up topics they think might be the motive for it and pass it on.

Don't be left behind on this rapid-paced lifestyles. Upgrade and live in the now.

## Chapter 3: Don't Stress

"Brain cells create thoughts; stress kills mind cells. Stress isn't a notable idea"

Dough hall.

What are we able to clearly get thru the use of stressing over matters? Nothing virtually, we simply dig the hole deeper and deeper and as we hold going, we input darkness.

Stressing over occasions in fact reasons a bigger mess of the state of affairs than it certainly is.

Getting worried if you have friends or site visitors coming over? Do your buddies surely determine you for the way you stay? Then permit me can help you recognise something,

There is not any shame in admitting you can't give you the coins for some thing. Anyone who judges you to your monetary situation doesn't deserve you.

If you're busy running and barely have the time to easy the residence it is first-class. No want to strain so much at the equal time as someone is about to go to and your house in now not in form. Just permit it's far. Stressing over such stuff really creates a larger problem.

What will take location while you try to easy the house in a hurry? You may moreover additionally grow to be knocking over some subjects left right here and there. You may be continuously angry or irritated. You might also shout at someone for something that doesn't even depend quantity. Sometimes family members of the own family are ruined in this way

Take a deep breath. Clean up on the pace you usually do. Do now not strain over being timebound.

If you aren't able to clean up on time, in truth make an apology. Everyone is busy nowadays, so it's in reality appropriate enough to be messy.

Many parents even though don't apprehend what we really need to aspire. We are out of place and don't apprehend what we really want to reap in life.

What if you haven't but determined on what you actually need to pursue. It will come to you eventually. There is lots to take a look at. Experience the pleasure of gaining knowledge of and training. Notice new topics. There isn't any want to hurry.

Another small problem of ours is that when our friends are busy taking area pricey holidays, we are walking difficult to make ends meet.

But why experience unhappy? Just due to the reality they have that costly, does no longer propose you don't have something in any respect in comparison to them. Maybe they might be going via some precise problems, which you are not and they may sense the identical looking at your lifestyles.

Just revel in wonderful. You can pull off any hardships!

"If some thing is bothering you, flow within the course of it rather than going for walks far from it."

Running away from your troubles isn't the proper answer.

Now how does stress play a issue in this? Well, we make small problems appearance big. How so? By stressing over them too much! Giving them the amount of interest they don't actually need.

If you may't do a tremendous element, don't do it. Simple! There's no need to pressure. When you acquire your actual self, you could understand and now not be ashamed, that there are a few belongings you aren't able to.

That character can and I can't. I hate the feel. That is a incorrect mind-set regarding situations.

"Your achievement and happiness lies in you. Resolve to keep your self happy, and your delight and also you shall form an invincible host against difficulties."

Helen Keller.

You can attain plenty. Don't ever count on you could't. You can. If you've got faith in yourself you may get via all of it. Just surround yourself with happiness and don't strain over topics.

Don't dig the hole deeper; instead cowl it up along facet your strength of thoughts and self guarantee.

When a automobile twist of future takes place, the air bag protects the passengers. You in fact can't forestall the crash, the damage accomplished to the car is performed, but the damage that might've been immoderate for the passenger, is forfeited to an extent.

Your faith in your self and your strength to overcome issues works the identical manner.

The damage finished to a degree is completed, so basically you may't inform the issues intending your manner to prevent, however you may cause them to lots a whole lot much less tough.

Respecting and accepting your right self. Don't be inexperienced with envy.

A brother and sister had contrasting abilties. The elder brother have become professional with numbers, at the equal time because the sister modified into correct at concept. She could not solve the perfect sum, but if you gave her a biology check, she may excel in it.

The sister become typically concerned that her grades have been falling simply due to her failure in math, whilst her brother managed to accumulate precise at concept as nicely.

Some days earlier than her final check she requested her brother to assist her out, so she ought to get some do better. Her brother began to educate her. He have grow to be devastated that his sister knew not anything! The sum he want to remedy in seconds should take her minutes to even apprehend the question.

But he did not get indignant at her, or make her feel that he is superior to her. Instead he taught her recommendations and made her apprehend the method the funny and smooth manner. She cherished analyzing maths and her examination went properly. Eventually the dad and mom had been satisfied that they did not wreck down due to the fact they have been willing somewhere. Rather they decided a manner out and revered each different's ability to do advantageous topics and not being able to perform a little.

What if the woman stopped attempting? She may want to no longer have been able to find out a solution for the trouble she changed into going via.

She idea attempting to find assist changed into better. She general her vulnerable point and decided she desired assist to overcome it.

She did not hesitate to definitely acquire her real self. Nor did she envy her brother. Her brother did now not criticize her for now not understanding easy math. He made her apprehend better, he knew she modified into modern in specific aspects.

She moved within the course of her problem and faced it.

LEARN TO LIVE ALONE AND BECOME INDEPENDENT

When we are pressured or stuck with a problem we attempting to find the assist of a person. A assisting hand, however you don't constantly get it.

That is why you need to be you. Have religion in yourself. Respect yourself. Bring out your personal slight, and shine vivid.

It's now not usually that you get a shoulder to lean on. People are not going to be there for you continuously. That's why you need to start managing matters on your private.

Become fearless, unique and make the right alternatives; you'll turn out to be independent.

Have you ever visited vintage age homes? We desire we had their expertise, right?

One of the vintage age houses I visit frequently is an area of surprise and understanding.

This one adorable and clumsy granny shared with me about what have come to be it that she regretted in existence. That isn't being capable of get knowledgeable and turn out to be independent. But education isn't always all that become needed to emerge as impartial.

She constantly asked me if I in truth have started out doing my very own artwork, started out making my non-public alternatives, trusting myself and standing up, now not excellent for myself, but for others too, if a scenario arose.

I modified into approximately to mutter a certain. I am unbiased you understand, but I changed into speechless.

Now I without a doubt marvel are anyone impartial? We ask our pals or circle of relatives members to head and purchase stuff for us or with us. When we get ill we are searching for the safe haven of our dad and mom and prevent functioning clearly!

When we ask our pals about how the trendy get dressed is and that they don't reply returned immediately, we start doubting ourselves. Do we plan a experience and get into considering such plenty of 'what if's' and genuinely cancel it? Funny,proper? So, we basically aren't unbiased.

Her purpose for asking the ones questions come to be her personal life enjoy of path. She had youngsters and she or he changed right into a housewife. Her husband changed into a mariner. They had been a middle-magnificence own family, however wealthier than their family. She did no longer have tons interest in getting informed but she went on have a have a examine till her 8th grade modified into finished. Well, in the ones times which have turn out to be a brilliant deal, particularly for a lady.

She modified into married off at the age of 25. The trouble she loved about her mother and father emerge as she may need to decide who she desires to marry .They never stopped her from learning. So she pursued a direction to investigate sewing and embroidery. Her mother and father additionally taught her to put together dinner. And yes, her dad cooked too! They made all of the siblings research the entirety. Vital capabilities of life are critical, they stated. Hence, her brother modified into taught a way to prepare dinner dinner too.

I am pointing this out because of the fact within the ones instances women were taken into consideration homely and boys have been the only to go out to work. Racist feedback had been continually there, but it have become no longer that horrible.

A year after her first infant turned into born; she became supplied an possibility to start a tailoring keep, considering the reality that she had the experience and statistics. Her husband did now not agree. And she did as have become informed. She denied the provide.

By the time her 2nd infant emerge as born, she started out out feeling lonely. Her husband became hardly ever home and he or she became all by myself to take care of them.

She stated "no one can say, oh I helped you beautify them. I raised my kids all on my own through thick and thin". But she did now not as soon as get desired for this. Her husband cared more for his family even after marriage. This bring about fights and over time they drifted apart.

"I could not live with out him nor need to he. But the accept as true with become now not the equal. It changed into damaged a long term inside the past" her voice and eyes depicted her ache.

"Emotions are in truth a top notch species I guess, however the early you discover your internal self and begin strolling on the aspect of your feelings, the better." This become what she anticipated me to do.

Later, as time went with the aid of manner of their own family suffered from economic issues. Her children understood even though. They in no manner complained approximately how they used to live a pretty lavish life and now they had to sacrifice plenty.

A best period arrived while she preferred to go away all of it. She used to cry because of the fact her husband blamed her and the children, however by no means ordinary his mistakes. She truely took it all because she desired her youngsters to get knowledgeable. At least he turn out to be paying for his or her training and that emerge as all she preferred.

The courage to certainly separate and start a current lifestyles; the normal fear for her kids and her earnings changed into taking a toll on her. She had really locked all the pain indoors herself. The husband started out announcing things like, "you don't earn, and I do. You do now not recognize how difficult it's miles." But did he ever understand how she modified into walking hard at domestic?

All this became hurting her masses. Eventually humans started out telling her this: 'you are in a miles better scenario, one-of-a-type housewives should have become abused you apprehend' and one-of-a-kind remarks have to comply with.

She may reply, "But what approximately my mind this is being abused and my coronary heart that feels discover it impossible to face up to's been punched?"

People say such subjects because of the reality they want you to sense higher. But the phrases hit her extra, it made her reckon that she became prone and making a huge fuss of such small issues.

She preferred to scream out that she become no longer prone. She changed into courageous and cared a lot for her infants.

She desired me to analyze a few problem from this tale of hers. Firstly, accept as actual collectively along with your instincts and stay your life passionately. If she had completed so, her tailoring artwork would have avoided future monetary troubles.

Secondly, she changed into grateful to her parents for training her the entirety, they in no manner pressured her for a few element, and they absolutely preferred her to in a feature to overcome the worst situations lifestyles threw at her. They treated all of the siblings with love and equality.

 Her dad and mom had been proud, she have end up sturdy enough to live by myself maximum of the time and lift her kids without a good buy of a help from all people. Then her youngsters have turn out to be her help tool.

So in no manner actually hate your dad and mom, they teach you for the higher.

And if any scenario arises, communicate it out. Don't lash out or make assumptions. You are part of them and they might in no way harm you. Their manner of showing love might be one-of-a-kind however they love you! So, it's miles better to talk and easy out the doubts.

Third, she knew her husband turn out to be wrong and so had been some of his family individuals, but she never really got the braveness to rebellion. She have become so stuck up inside the feelings. She modified into involved about what may additionally appear 'if' this and 'if' that. She perplexed what if she had walked out and actually began out out over? She need to have commenced small after which made it large. She had her brother's assist too. She lost an possibility.

Fourth, she held expectancies. She idea the praises can also help enhance her ego, however that is what backfired. When her expectations had been broken, she modified into harm.

We in the first vicinity make assumptions and recall such lovable situations that we're broken while matters don't pass as in keeping with our thoughts. We end up crying.

Stop having expectations. Even while a person ensures a component; do now not keep directly to it, count on the greater intense. So despite the fact that topics go with the flow wrong by one percentage, you will be organized for it.

Fifth, she knew why people had been announcing such matters, however at the inner, she started out out out questioning too much and ended up blaming herself for the activities.

She had misplaced herself and he or she preferred the antique her lower once more. It modified into now not too late, she advanced. She commenced wondering, that irrespective of what, she might be pleased with herself. Proud of what she is these days. Proud of wherein is now.

It does no longer do not forget amount if humans don't see or understand what she did. She knew what she did and that become all that changed into preferred. Born on my own, die on my own with none regrets.

She began out to reduce out the memories of her past and sulking over why she did not take a choice. The time has passed and he or she or he needed to attention on the prevailing, at the contemporary-day-day 2nd what need to she do? How can also want to she make subjects better and live inside the 2nd to make all of it properly well really worth?

She used to recognition on her husband's fascinating factors, so that she won't hurt.

So now how independent are you in reality? How a long way are you able to bypass by myself?

I recognize there are various matters we need help with. But we need to make ourselves tough. Remember the manner you need to stand the problem and flow within the direction of it as opposed to on foot a long way from it. Troubles aren't something to be not noted.

Always endure in thoughts, no character has a small or huge trouble. The damage completed to the brain can't be visible physically, but it hurts the same manner. Failing to understand that, is the error every body devote.

Just like how the cuts want to be bandaged, our mind desires to be dealt with. We want to fill it with positivity and brace ourselves for the worst. Even in case you sense low, do no longer stress. Just be calm. Think. And do what you need to do. Find tactics you could deal with subjects, be sincere and you shall be triumphant.

## Chapter 4: Learn To Forgive

Do you continue to preserve grudges in competition to someone? Or you absolutely sense like hitting a person terrible?

Why can we start to hate? Now a days humans begin selecting up fights for no cause.

We need to be there for others. I recognize we stated how we need to be unbiased, and how we need to be there for every exceptional.

You need to be there however furthermore be prepared on the same time as someone is not there. They are particular times.

Start forgiving. It will result in a trade in you. When we see a person with whom we as soon as had awful instances brings back the memories of hate. We do not want that. Humans commit mistakes, all people does and we want to forgive.

Some phrases spoken by means of someone can't be forgiven, but keep in mind at the same time as you dedicate a mistake, you pray for forgiveness. You pray to him just so he can wash away your sins. Maybe the character dreams the identical and in case you forgive them, you bypass on a active message to them.

Strength, an trouble we were speaking about, to grow to be unbiased – forgiveness performs an vital feature in it. You add on power the day you discover ways to forgive.

Forgiving and trusting again is some other tale. You just need to overlook what took place however have a take a look at now not to get related once more.

The case of the vintage woman proper here, she learnt to forgive her husband, to hold the peace among her families. But the actual do not forget became broken and it could not be mended lower back.

We need to create peace. Peace is what makes the region a glad location.

## DON'T BE UP IN YOUR HEAD; BE IN THE PRESENT AND STAY CONNECTED TO IT

To take hold of the possibility, you need to be capable enough to be aware it and make the most of it.

To be up for your head essentially technique, you determined you are definitely residing the existing and making the maximum of it however you virtually are definitely making it all up for your head and now not truly searching at and functioning inside the now.

Stories are the fine manner to portray a message, so right proper here is going each unique one.

Once, a professor and a pupil determined to go on a adventure as a damage from the hustle of existence. After a long adventure, the professor commenced feeling thirsty.

But they were inside the center of a large farmland with an empty bottle. They could not discover any supply of water, until the professor observed a small hut a mile earlier. They walked closer to it in the choice that they may simply find out a person who might be capable of quench their thirst.

Hopefully as they neared the gate of the hut a man walked out have come to be greater than inclined to offer them water and some snack. While they have been having a communicate, the professor requested the man or woman "How do you live on in this enormous land?" The guy spoke back, "I very very very own a cow and via promoting its milk and ghee made with none adulteration, we suffice." Then the professor questioned, "do you non-public this land, all of it till that mountain's boundary?" the man nodded a sure proudly. The professor had doubts so he confused him all over again, "But then why don't you grow vegetables proper right here, you'll be a farmer" the person chuckled and replied, "But who desires that for? We can stay with this, that is genuinely enough; our youngsters also are used to living like this."

The debate ended there and the professor determined to stay the night, the person changed into extra than satisfied to have web site traffic.

At midnight the professor woke his scholar up and requested him to comply with. The student became forced. Where did he need to move at this hour? He quietly followed his professor and as soon as they observed the cow, the professor counseled the student to tie him loose and follow him. The student have come to be baffled, what have grow to be taking area? But he dared now not query him and quietly observed. As they reached the border of the farmland, the professor set the cow free, and driven it within the other direction. The student in the end asked what modified into he doing this for? What will display as much as the cow and the man? It turned into his splendid technique of earning.

The professor suggested him not to worry and get once more to sleep.

Early subsequent morning, they took their depart. The guy had not however notices his missing cow.

After some years, the professor contacted his student and asked him to accompany him for a journey all yet again. The student gladly popular and that they left the following morning.

The scholar changed into amazed to look his professor taking him to the identical farmland where they spent a night time, long term in the past. What surprised him greater emerge as that the location come to be now not the identical. There changed into greenery all around and as opposed to a hut there was a cemented residence, which changed into larger than the hut.

The man of the house walked out to see who modified into traveling and the professor greeted the person and requested if he remembered them but the guy furrowed his eyebrows, mumbling "Sorry. No."

The professor elaborated how that they'd visited one night thirsty at his region and he allow them to stay the night time too.

The man smiled, "Yes I do now. The pupil and the professor."

The pupil changed into satisfied that the man or woman cited them and he asked "How did this all exchange? You are clearly farming and this vicinity appears greener and in addition stunning."

"Yes son, surely the day you guys left, our cow had all of sudden disappeared. We did no longer have something else, so we started slowly with the resource of developing some vegetables and staples. Then we supplied some other cow, but my own family genuinely loved farming, so we endured."

"That's actually specific!" The student smiled big.

"Yes. It is. We even export the cease quit result and a few vegetables." The guy modified into feeling proud.

After the professor and scholar had tea, they took their go away.

The professor defined to his student why he did that years within the beyond.

"If we wouldn't have accomplished that he might likely nevertheless be the equal, stuck up in his head. Now that the outcomes changed, he modified too. So, on occasion, you need to do wrong to make the some thing right."

The student nodded in settlement, "But you understand I revel in horrific for the cow." he frowned.

"Don't want to, I had some guys pass take him to the cow secure haven. Not extremely good that specific one, however additionally some others who have been now not in an splendid form. I now send charge variety for them and the high-quality that belonged to this man has been introduced all once more and is happy."

"You acquired not anything from that man in favour of what you probably did for him and he's despite the fact that unaware that we untied his cow and he did not honestly set himself free."

"Don't worry, you have a look at with time. I did now not have expectancies. I did no longer do it to accumulate compliments; I did it for the destiny technology. Helping someone in want is an instinct.

## Chapter 5: Conquer Addictions

The first dependancy this is going to pop in everybody's thoughts is smoking and consuming.

And this is true. Because, quite some teenagers are hooked on the ones dangerous topics.

Smoking is terrible for our fitness. Tobacco is volatile.

Drinking is okay to some extent. Then we come to the class of medication which humans get hooked on.

But these are not the only addictions.

Excess of a few aspect is in no manner pinnacle. There are other varieties of dependancy too- Internet, Plastic surgical operation, purchasing, telephones, apps and loads extra.

These days anybody desires to get excessive. Not first-class teenagers additionally adults, they need to overlook approximately approximately their issues and do some element that distracts them and makes them experience satisfied. Then they turn to tablets.

But as we said earlier than, excess of something is dangerous.

To escape from the hustle bustle of towns, we circulate for a journey to the united states of the us facet. But it's uncommon. We don't adventure backward and forward each day.

We are aware about it's all incorrect but additionally a lot amusing, so we grow to be focusing at the fun element and start neglecting the incorrect that it brings along.

Stop yourself from falling in too deep.

If you are addicted, get keep of it. Do no longer hesitate to are seeking out for help, you obtained't be judged.

A person getting addicted might also additionally have one-of-a-type motives for it and we want to understand that. If you aren't addicted, but apprehend a person who is, assist them.

Don't lash without delay to human beings for being hooked on some factor. Try to apprehend their motive for beginning some component. They is probably compelled or sincerely having a bad time.

Smokers need to forget about their issues. That's why they smoke. Some cannot nod off due to the fact their mind is type of a storm. So they drink till they doze off. When such matters assist them, they simply get addicted to it. It starts offevolved from a addiction and movements directly to a compulsion.

You need to attain out and help. There's a manner to each hassle.

Sometimes it's now not pretty tons attempting, liking it and getting addicted.

Our thoughts works in another way. We certainly start yearning and before we realize it, we exit of manipulate.

So, do not hesitate, be strong and confident. Conquer your addictions and also you'll be relieved.

Don't surrender although it is hard. Keep reminding your self that you aren't a quitter and also you obtained't surrender. Believe that there are proper times in advance. Believe that you may get out of your problems. Believe within the present.

MEDITATE AND EXERCISE

Meditation and everyday exercising are crucial for a wholesome way of life.

They are your mood busters and effective for preventing despair.

Meditation turns on the parasympathetic anxious system, which reduces strain reaction. That isn't the handiest benefit. If you are continuously meditating, it permits you discover ways to recognize your very personal mind. The manner mind come and bypass. It adjustments the thoughts in an exceptional way.

Exercising permits preserve your frame in form, moreover allows you distract your self from issues, makes you feel free and boosts yourself perception.

You do no longer must constantly join a health club to workout. You simply need to awaken and meditate. Then indulge yourself in a few yoga and exercise.

Yoga allows remedy many diseases and one-of-a-type sorts of frame aches. It makes you bendy. Yoga in truth holds a completely unique energy inside.

The calmer and focused you emerge as, the more you may able to live in the now. Your attention electricity will increase. When you indulge your self in such sports activities you'll forget about your concerns.

You can attend dance commands. There isn't always any rule that during case you want to turn out to be a dancer pleasant then you definately have the proper to enroll in a dance elegance. It permits you live fit .And what's a better combination than music and a few body moves to permit all that pressure out!?

Whatever making a decision upon, begin from these days itself! It's in no manner too late to begin training an amazing addiction.

## Chapter 6: What Is Mindfulness?

Mindfulness is the act of preserving an lively and open reputation on our frame, feelings, environment, and thoughts. Being conscious permits an individual to intentionally discern one's emotions, thoughts, and feelings with out effects considering them to be accurate or awful. Mindfulness lets in an person to truely stay in the 2d rather than allowing existence to virtually bypass them with the useful resource of. When you are in a kingdom of being conscious, you generally have a tendency to experience the instant and neglect about to brood about the beyond nor good buy or reckon at the destiny.

The time period mindfulness came from the time period sati of the Pali, a language native to the Indians. Sati is an essential element in Buddhist traditions. Mindfulness has completed a detail too in Buddhist traditions. Buddhists exercising mindfulness to domesticate know-how and self-data will step-thru-step, result in what is thought of getting a whole freedom from pain or enlightenment.

Mindfulness has come to be well-known as nicely within the America for the beyond years and Jon Kabat-Zinn is in element answerable for it. He is concept to be the brain of the Mindfulness-Based Stress Reduction or MBSR which changed into added in 1979 on the University of Massachusetts Medical School. A quantity of studies had been documented concerning the mental and bodily health advantages of mindfulness thinking about that then. The Mindfulness -Based Stress Reduction has inspired a persevering with listing of programs to adapt its very personal version for colleges, hospitals, veteran centers, and prisons to name a few.

More so, Jon Kabat-Zinn also gave a proof on how mindfulness triggers some part of an man or woman's mind which aren't usually energetic at the equal time as one is on autopilot mode mindlessly.

Mindfulness has considering been used to assist mother and father which might be experiencing exclusive forms of mental issues. Various recuperation programs based mostly on mindfulness have furthermore been superior. Here are some of the highbrow ailments in which mindfulness is being used: treatment of drug addiction, lessening anxiety, decreasing strain, and diminishing signs and signs and symptoms and signs of despair Practicing the art work of mindfulness offers the have an effect on of handing over some of therapeutic advantages to human beings with psychosis. It additionally can be used as a preventive method to save you the development of various further highbrow health troubles.

Another mindfulness guru, Steven Hick, says that the exercise of mindfulness is comprised of each formal and informal meditation practices. Nonmeditation-primarily based completely carrying sports also are involved inside the mindfulness exercise.

According to him, mindfulness is classified into : Formal and casual. Formal mindfulness, also called meditation, is the workout of withstanding interest on sensations, body, or a few element that pretty plenty floor in each 2d. Informal mindfulness, however, is the software of conscious hobby in a unmarried's very own regular lifestyles.

How Mindfulness Started

Mindfulness is notion to be a custom engaged with exceptional religious and nonreligious praxis, from Hinduism and Buddhism to yoga and, all the more as of overdue, non-spiritual mirrored image. Through the years, a number of humans have been utilising mindfulness in their everyday lives, regardless of whether or not or not independent from all and sundry else or as a feature of a bigger custom.

It has been identified that mindfulness changed into made well-known within the primary within the East and non secular and spiritual corporations are a good deal answerable for it. On the alternative hand, mindfulness grow to be recognized inside the West thru the efforts of some precise human beings and extraordinary temporal groups.

Fact is, even the non-religious way of life of mindfulness in the West owes its foundations to the Eastern religion or even to specific practitioners of Eastern religions.

Although mindfulness is lots regarded to have its roots in Buddhism and Hinduism, it furthermore has its roots in Judaism, Islam, and Christianity.

From East to West

Jon Kabat-Zinn became already stated on the primary a part of this ebook. However, it won't be not possible now not to say him again and again all at some point of this ebook as every person realize that he is the most vital have an impact on on the equal time as said how mindfulness has unfold its affect from the East to the West.

This well-known influencer of mindfulness is the founding father of the Center for Mindfulness stationed at the University of Massachusetts Medical School and the Oasis Institute for Mindfulness-Based Professional Education and Training. In this foundation is wherein the incredible mindfulness guru has advanced his Mindfulness-Based Stress Reduction software or moreover called MBSR.

The Mindfulness-Based Stress Reduction software is an eight-week software program program which motive is to reduce an person's degrees of pressure.

Thich Nhat Hanh, a famous and an influential discern in Western mindfulness, and extraordinary severa Buddhist teachers, are the influencers of Jon Kabat-Zinn at the same time as he have become analyzing and learning more of the paintings of mindfulness. Combining the subjects he found out from them and with Western technological know-how, he have become capable of increase the Mindfulness-Based Stress Reduction software. The MBSR is an important attempt in helping mindfulness advantage incredible popularity within the West.

The MBSR program crammed in as a motivation for some different care primarily based absolutely remedy software program, it really is the Mindfulness-Based Cognitive Therapy (MBCT). This treatment's goal is to treat Major Depressive Disorder.

## Chapter 7: Mindfulness Plus Psychology

Mindfulness assumes a crucial component in each the extra outstanding location of mind studies and powerful mind technology specifically. MBSR and MBCT have grew to come to be out to be mentioned units for therapists to address an series of sufferers with, demonstrating the benefit of mindfulness lessons in traditional brain research. With recognize to powerful psychology, mindfulness has turn out to be a useful tool for everyone hoping to construct their tiers of prosperity, and MBSR has moreover grew to become out to be wonderful in non-scientific populations.

Some can also furthermore even say that psychology and its tremendous have at ultimate all commenced to recognize mindfulness in a way that Eastern customs have appeared for millenia. Specifically, Western technological know-how has now superior to the component in which it could determine the viability of working within the path of mindfulness, making it an appealing opportunity for the folks who are doubtful of Eastern customs for one-of-a-kind motives.

Mindfulness Plus Philosophy

The workout of mindfulness may additionally additionally need to indicate a yoga exercise that consists of mindfulness. In can include making time for mindfulness meditation training or working towards it in the course of one's every day activities like washing the dishes and so forth.

Mindfulness is a no sweat exercise. Anyone can do it and there are various exceptional mindfulness sports activities which can be performed. These activities may be practiced to come to be more mindful and there also are a number of mindfulness practices and groups which are particularly designed for precise corporations of people.

Regardless, of your identification or what your every day lifestyles carries of, there can be in all threat a mindfulness exercise customized to you. This flexibility makes it open to all who will examine and placed only a bit of a time in. This is a critical piece of the philosophy, no matter whether or now not it's miles rehearsed religiously or in a nonreligious way. All matters taken into consideration, individuals who workout mindfulness are, for the maximum component taking a shot at a comparable problem, regardless of whether or not or no longer they call it careful mindfulness or edification, and now not very many (assuming any) mindfulness depend upon confining their instructions to a sole bracket.

Why Should You Practice Mindfulness?

Now that you already have an concept what mindfulness is, you is probably thinking why it has emerge as a mainstream treatment or why it is been pointed out through the usage of plenty of human beings from pretty an awful lot anywhere.

Anyone can exercise mindfulness, it comes obviously for each person in any form which encompass meditation, yoga, or actually via virtually taking a 2d to pause and breathe while doing any shape of duties in preference to speeding via just to have it finished.

When we method our lives mindfully, we have were given were given a famous feeling of stepped forward mindfulness, quietness and physical unwinding. These are absolutely sizeable motivations to exercise mindfulness, but the advantages go an extended tactics beyond that.

There is a list of motives why one must workout mindfulness. Here's a rundown of it.

Mindfulness builds up bodily health. Scientists have determined that the benefits of sure mindfulness strategies help one beautify his/her physical fitness in a number of approaches.

Mindfulness develops properly-being. Being aware makes an man or woman without issues experience the pleasures in existence as they seem inside the intervening time and allows you to be absolutely concerned in great sports activities sports. Since one is capable of attention on the here and now, quite a few folks who exercise mindfulness discover themselves less probable to fear about the destiny and neglect about about the regrets they've got in the beyond. More so, they tend to be lots much less preoccupied with apprehensions approximately vanity and achievement, making them more approachable and letting them form deep connections with others.

Mindfulness betters intellectual fitness. Mindfulness meditation has thinking about that been treated with the aid of psychotherapists as an critical element of treatment of various intellectual and nonpsychological troubles collectively with the subsequent:

-Anxiety problems

-Couples' conflicts

-Depression

-Drug abuse

-Eating issues

-Obsessive-compulsive disorder

Lessens Stress. Mindfulness is taken into consideration to be an crucial element in reducing strain. According to Howden and Medibank, these are a number of the symptoms and symptoms of strain:

-Constantly feeling traumatic and concerned

-Feeling irritable, agitated, and without hassle irritated

-Argumentative and shielding with buddies and family

-Restless snoozing

-Low degrees of strength, regularly waking up feeling worn-out

-Restless and frenetic mind

-Often self-essential and/or critical of others

-Feeling flat and uninspired

-Having problem concentrating

-Skin rashes and situations

-Clenching your jaw muscle tissue and grinding your enamel at night time time time

-Headaches and migraines

These signs and signs and symptoms and signs and symptoms of strain may be diminished or better, relieved even as one practices mindfulness. By workout mindfulness, you are able to gain a country of relaxation, therefore, acquiring this listing of blessings:

-Amplified clarity in questioning and notion

-Boosted hobby and recognition

-Better immune gadget

-Built-up recognition

-Increased brain feature

-Lowered blood stress

-Reduced tension stages

-Feel the sensation of being calm and internally nonetheless

-Undergo the feeling of being related

The listing of blessings goes on and also you'll get greater of those by truly ultimate your eyes and be silent for just for a couple of minutes an afternoon. Anyone can do it as it's smooth as 1-2-three!

## Chapter 8: Lessen Symptoms Of Depression

Depression is one of the maximum continual highbrow infection nowadays, and it is also one of the most commonplace ones. It is said that as an entire lot as 80 percent of the folks who go through a large time depressive stage may additionally moreover moreover relapse despite the fact that below the have an impact on of medicinal capsules. With this situation, numerous studies has been made to success the warfare toward despair.

One of the answers decided is schooling mindfulness – in particular the usage of the MBCT. The MBCT program have turn out to be said to as powerful as taking safety antidepressant medicinal tablets.

Mindfulness-Based Cognitive Therapy (MBCT) is being applied to help stop melancholy relapse. It consolidates intellectual conduct systems with mindfulness strategies which encompass meditation and breathing activities to assist exchange the cycle of horrible mind regular with periodic melancholy. The Mindfulness-Based Cognitive Therapy generally consists of 8 week- after-week, two-hour mixture academic publications, normal homework assignments, and observe-up gatherings. Home assignments may additionally furthermore include mindfulness activities and work on coordinating mindfulness abilities into every day life. A current-day meta-analysis taking a gander at mindfulness-based definitely subjective treatment used to assist keep away from depression relapse and idea that it changed into a fulfillment, especially for sufferers with greater excessive state of affairs.

One of the techniques wherein mindfulness can help deal with despair is thru enhancing professionals' capability to manipulate their emotions. Mindfulness offers the system expected to assignment over again from intense horrific feelings, distinguish them, and widely recognized them in vicinity of scuffling with them. This method allows aware masterminds to higher direct their emotions, prompting higher adapting and dealing with despair.

Improved Academic Success for Kids and Students

Andy does not clearly excel properly academically. Her grades are constantly low ever for the purpose that she became in High School. She has tried tutors, all-nighter studying, organization research, man or woman studies, name it. She technically di nearly a few component truely to improve her academic grades. But however all of the effort she stored on exerting, it genuinely does no longer seem to paintings. She came at some point of a piece of writing on mindfulness in the end and determined out how mindfulness can do the trick in searching for to excel in college, and bet what? It virtually labored!

Various research show that mindfulness has performed a massive characteristic in enhancing a toddler's academic fulfillment.

A examine via manner of Harpin, Rossi, Kim, & Swanson, 2016 showed that simple college students who practiced mindfulness confirmed more prosocial behaviors, emotion law, and advanced educational universal performance. This have a study is in addition greater superb with a have a study thru Bennett & Dorjee, 2016 which resulted that teens who took element in a mindfulness software skilled lesser despair and tension which in the end contributed in their superior instructional attainment.

Here are extra studies to decrease again up the efficiency of mindfulness to a student's educational success.

•A take a look at thru Viafora, Mathiesen, & Unsworth, 2015 confirmed that homeless middle university college students who participated in a mindfulness route confirmed better well-being which could cause a fantastic educational success and ensuing to a much higher top notch of lifestyles

•Sibinga, Perry-Parrish, Chung, Johnson, Smith & Ellen, 2013 look at shows that inside the MBSR carried out on city male young people, those male youths skilled a lesser quantity of tension, negativity, and stress, which reason their functionality to decorate their functionality to address the pressure brought thru academics and accomplishing better college grades.

•Costello & Lawler, 2014 carried out a look at that showed that children from lower socioeconomic backgrounds who participated in a 5-week mindfulness software advocated decreased strain, letting them focus on college

Mindfulness Can Help Stand Up Against Bullying

Charles has normally been a sufferer of their campus. Being a Grade 8 student, skinny, wears glasses, and an introvert, he has always been the only being picked on. It emerge as no longer normally that way. He had friends once more then. Unfortunately, his buddies each moved out or determined a person way cooler than him, because of this, giving bullies extra motives to pick on him. He maintains pretending to be used with all of the bullying, but human as he is, he's despite the fact that liable to the mental and emotional results bullying brings him. But that is not the case now, mindfulness has helped him cope up with all of the bullying.

A column with the resource of manner of Houlihan from the University of Massachusetts at Boston states that "Mindfulness practices help the bully, sufferer, and any witnesses worried develop a deeper awareness of themselves, resilience, compassion, and a greater capability to regulate their emotional responses,"

Mindfulness programs are starting to be carried out for a few schools those packages should in all likelihood reduce the impact that bullying need to strong on sufferers and the majority of the school community.

Mindfulness can also have an effect on bullies. Fear of being the distinct one, having low vanity, depressing situation at home - the ones are definitely some of the problems a bully has and people are just some of what drives them to end up one. So how does mindfulness does play its feature on this?

Mindfulness can reach to the very center of what pushes the bullying conduct within the first vicinity. It can also educate bullies and others a way to end up more empathetic of others, for this reason reducing the urge to bully and the instances of bullying.

More so, mindfulness boosts vanity, and for the reason that having low conceitedness is one of the troubles of a bully person, it is able to create an development. Having boosted self guarantee can decrease the opportunity of bullying with the useful useful resource of making perpetrators be greater snug of their non-public individuality - lessening the need of compelled approval and recognize from others.

Mindfulness Can Provide Support and Boost Resilience

When humans are pressured, challenged, and/or need to accept a exchange in their each day routine or so, strain genuinely abruptly kicks in for max, as a consequence making them more irritable. When such incident continues, it could give up result to tension or despair.

Resilience is what people want to workout in a few unspecified time within the future of those activities. Resilience is the capability to react properly to difficulty and it may help keep one's positivity, adaptability, and higher thoughts-set while strain really kicks in.

Mindfulness education may be the critical factor to boost, beautify, and gather the resilience humans want.

## Chapter 9: Awareness

Complaining approximately top notch subjects is not a super dependancy, however we exercising it intentionally or no longer. It can create an impact on an man or woman's intellectual well-being, physical health, courting with others, and their mood.

Mindfulness furthermore teaches people the "Appreciative Awareness" wherein they are taught on appreciating a few subjects even if things get tough.

This technique from mindfulness permits humans increase their self guarantee, end up healthy, live fantastic, and be more resilient.

Keeping Healthy Relationships

Mindfulness lets in an individual to create and preserve amazing relationships with others the usage of quite a few procedures. Through it, an individual is given time to assume or pause for some time, making her or him heaps less probable to create a judgement and blurt it out of anger or out of other bad moods she or he has within the suggest time. It will reduce or eliminate a experience of regret at the same time as a few detail impolite is stated simply because of the truth judgements have been no longer idea thru.

Relationships are crucial to gather resilience. It will permit you to stay robust sincerely via putting in as masses as a person who cares about you.

Problem Solving

Using mindfulness, an individual may have a more widespread interest which then effects to a greater open and new possibilities and connections. When an character is in a kingdom of mindfulness, his or her prefrontal cortex is surely lively.

Stress Response

Mindfulness lets in the mind to react distinctively to pressure. It physical makes the amygdala smaller, making the individual much less willing to the fight-flight response. That implies they're capable of stay take a seat lower back, quiet and amassed beneath a large quantity of pressure. They normally tend to have decrease blood stress and a far advanced immune device which makes them masses wholesome and masses less liable to ailments

## Mindfulness Can Reduce Work-Related Stress and Distress

In present day rapid-phasing global, especially on workplaces, personnel are faced with a exceptional lis of duties, dreams, and annoying conditions which frequently makes one pressured. This strain because of superb factors from the place of business can also end result to declining effeciancy, effectiveness, and creativity - extra so, on how they address the humans round their working environment. These can reason increased worker absences and reduced productiveness.

With those issues that stand up on offices, employers and/or HR human beings motel to the mindfulness exercising for his or her employees as it boosts stress management and promotes self-take care of the personnel. The mindfulness practice moreover allows employees to be greater powerful in communique and create a more exquisite working dating amongst others.

It we may need to us get to recognise our genuine self

Mindfulness triggers individuals to supply out their "watching self". The "searching at self " is idea to be part of an character that is natural awareness. It allows one to take phrase of everything that she or he does, assume, revel in, and say.

It supports your weight loss desires

Losing weight can be a task for some people. There are numerous strategies to collect the weight they desire, but proper right here's an underrated possibility to conducting your weight aim: mindfulness.

More and similarly human beings now end result to operating towards mindfulness to reap their preferred weight. Through mindfulness, humans will be inclined to devour their food in a much slower and thoughtful way, plus figuring out whether or now not they need to munch on processed and horrific food or pick out out the plenty healthful preference.

Mindful consuming, as it's miles recognized makes an person be conscious of the scent, flavor, heady scent, texture, and the colour of the meals they may be approximately to ear. It moreover permits the character to exercise chewing his or her food slowly and removing distractions at the equal time as consuming like reading or looking the television. It is understood that getting distracted with one among a type sports even as consuming may moreover slow down or stop the digestion of food.

There are numerous aware consuming techniques which might be practiced in recent times. Some of those conscious ingesting techniques are believed to resource in treating eating problems and of route, assist with weight reduction issues.

Mindfulness makes individuals eat an awful lot extra healthful food making it feasible to shed kilos even without utilizing numerous diet strategies. It moreover lets in decrease the urge to eat a few trouble an character quite an lousy lot craves for.

It allows you sleep better

Admit it, sleep is crucial for each one people. It allows to eventually have a clearly needed relaxation all of us deserves. But what in case you're one of the unlucky some who suffers from insomnia or any sort of infection while you may get an excellent night time's sleep for that depend?

Some can also moreover inn to snoozing pills, some depend upon analyzing books, others may select out the old skool manner – counting sheep. Well, is that approach in truth powerful? Nonetheless, with all of the strategies an person can try to help himself or herself fall to sleep, a few however hotel to mindfulness.

Aware now of what mindfulness can do to an individual gives a touch on how it could assist an character sleep better. Practicing mindfulness each day or for just even a few minutes in advance than drowsing can bring one's thoughts into interest of one's personal thoughts, emotions, sensations, and feelings. When this takes place, the character then can control them higher in preference to permitting them to take over him or her.

A quantity of scientific studies indicates that mindfulness allows in overcoming severa issues – issues that still consists of stress and includes sleep disturbance and tension that leads to melancholy.

When one practices mindfulness in advance than sleeping through meditation or actually taking time to breathe and loosen up, an tremendous night time time's sleep will soon look at.

Mindfulness Practices

A few varieties of meditation basically embody fixation—rehashing an expression or concentrating at the affect of respiratory, permitting the parade of mind that during reality emerge to transport backward and forward. Focus reflected photograph systems, and in addition splendid physical video video games, for example, jujitsu or yoga, can set off the super unwinding reaction, it's miles as a substitute profitable in diminishing the frame's response to strain.

According to helpguide.Org, mindfulness meditation builds upon interest practices. Here's the way it works:

• Go with the glide. In mindfulness meditation, after you installation consciousness, you check the float of inner mind, feelings, and bodily sensations without judging them as exact or terrible.

• Pay interest. You moreover be aware external sensations which include sounds, attractions, and contact that make up your 2d-to-2d experience. The project isn't to latch onto a selected concept, emotion, or sensation, or to get stuck in considering the past or the destiny. Instead you watch what comes and is going on your thoughts, and discover which intellectual conduct produce a feeling of properly-being or struggling.

• Stay with it. At instances, this manner won't seem enjoyable in any respect, however over time it gives a key to extra happiness and self-awareness as you turn out to be comfortable with a miles wider and wider form of your critiques.

One must moreover workout popularity. Accepting anything all of sudden comes all of a sudden on the triumphing 2nd. An character, whilst running towards mindfulness, could be type and forgiving of himself or herself at some stage in any scenario.

If you discover your self daydreaming, making plans, or criticizing, try to take phrase in which it leads and wherein it has lengthy past and carefully direct it for your sensations inside the present. Simply start over again if you bypass over an supposed meditation session.

This interest suggests crucial care contemplation.

Sit on a right away-upheld seat or with folded legs on the floor.

Concentrate on a part of your breathing, as an example, the impressions of air streaming into your nostrils and out of your mouth, or your tummy developing and falling as you breathe in and breathe out.

Once you have got were given confined your fixation alongside the ones strains, start to amplify your middle hobby. End up naturally conscious of sounds, sensations, and your mind.

Grasp and recollect each idea or sensation without passing judgment on it brilliant or awful. On the off risk that your thoughts begins offevolved to race, repair your attention to your fun. At that point growth your mindfulness all over again.

A less formal manner to address mindfulness can likewise will let you remain inside the gift and virtually to take an hobby for your existence. You can choose out any venture or minute to hone informal mindfulness, regardless of whether or not or not you're consuming, showering, taking walks, touching an partner, or playing with a tyke or grandchild. Taking care of those focuses will offer help:

•Begin by means of the usage of obtaining your regard for the sensations your body

•Take in thru your nostril, permitting the air descending into your lower paunch. Give your guts a risk to growth really.

•Next,inhale out through your mouth

•Notice the impressions of every inward breath and exhalation

•Continue with the excercise needing to be performed steadily and with full attention

•Connect in conjunction with your senses virtually. Notice each sight, contact, and sound with the motive that you revel in each sensation.

When you notice that your thoughts has meandered from the hobby wanting to be completed, tenderly take your interest lower back to the vibes gift other than the whole thing else.

## Chapter 10: 3-Way Mindfulness Habits For The Morning

How we upward push up within the morning basically influences how some thing remains of the day unfurls. There are a couple of things we're able to comprise into our first mild table which can have a brief impact in helping us in being more careful, self-humane, associated, and flexible in the route of the day.

Put your judgments apart and try those out completed the following week as an exam... allow your experience to be your manual.

1. Organize Your First Sounds: Rather than beginning the vacation day with an alert that affects your body to stressful and be startled, choose out an alert this is touchy and mitigating—tolls, chimes, all of the more unwinding track, some aspect it can be. This permits your frame to soak up a few thing relieving to begin the day.

2. Hydrate Before You Caffeinate: Rather than going straight away for the coffee or tea, check whether or now not or now not you could absorb a super glass of water. Your body is have been given dried out— your frame dreams water, it hasn't drank water during the night time. At that aspect waft in your espresso or tea.

3. Watch Nature: Instead of getting your innovation within the first region, flow into outdoor and take within the sky, take in a tree—permit your eyes and frame to take that in. At that detail maintain onward to beginning your day.

Mindfulness in Three Minutes

The 3-Minute Breathing Space (3MBS) is a schooling that is one of the more solid practices within the 8-week Mindfulness-Based Cognitive Therapy Program. Individuals say they recognize it. They assume that it's miles treasured. What's more, it has moreover superior into outstanding projects which are covered with mental nicely-being, management, practise, and extraordinary circles of lifestyles.

The 3-Minute Breathing Space

In the initial step of the 3MBS, the bait is to accumulate thoughtfulness concerning our enjoy to a extra tremendous and greater open manner that isn't normally required with selecting or deciding on or assessing, but certainly retaining—turning into a compartment for contemplations sentiments or sensations within the body which may be to be had and checking whether or no longer or not we're in a position to watch them, starting with one minute then onto the following. So a widescreen on which a full-size variety of factors can pop up.

In the second step, we are solicited to give up from that widescreen and to carry a interest this is significantly more idea and focused, so smaller, on taking in a unmarried locale of our our our bodies—the breath of the stomach, or the chest, or the nostrils, or wherever that the breath makes itself known, and keeping that more centered center hobby. So the eye right here is restricted, in contrast to the substantial technique inside the first step.

In the 1/3 step, at the same time as we pass out to wind up it seems that clearly conscious of sensations within the body all in all, sitting with the complete frame, the complete breath, once more, we circulate once more to greater extremely good and open compartment of consideration for our enjoy.

So what precisely is going in advance in the 3MBS. At one degree, if you're amidst a programmed, or multitasking minute, there's an area that you can skip your psyche that lets in you to decorate out of these schedules and the requests they located on our attention. Essentially, taking a seat and permitting your regard for skip in these numerous techniques may be very treasured in the end of the day.

In any case, what exactly is going ahead with our attention? The 3MBS as we've were given composed is really a awesome deal about shifting attention mainly methods to permit us to free ourselves or to get unstuck from a number of the ones programmed schedules.

In the space of spherical three mins we pass from huge, to restriction, to big yet again.

This takes place within the format, on the off danger that you can of a hourglass, which can be viewed as having a tremendous taking off, a truely restriction neck, and a large base.

These are analogies to depict the improvement of interest. What's extra, the development of interest is some component that I get preserve of is in truth useful about the 3MBS. Since whilst we're determined in multitasking, or programmed schedules, regularly our attention is not typically available to us, and it's miles not by using the usage of any stretch of the creativeness being guided or coordinated with the useful resource of our deliberateness.

Mindfulness vs Anger

Outrage—it has a appropriate strength. Simply bear in mind the ultimate time you honestly felt it. What phrases strike a chord? Hot? Adrenaline surge?

We're now not sure to react to outrage a comparable manner on every occasion we revel in it. By taking gain of the revel in of concern, and conveying empathy to it, we are able to determine out how to method this perilous, often risky feeling healthierly.

Bring round 3 minutes with each response. You may additionally additionally furthermore likewise increase that point at the off threat that you want to strive extra electricity.

1. Sit in an agreeable but ready feature collectively along with your palms resting effortlessly and your eyes delicately close to. Check in at the side of your body, and revel in the spots in which it reaches the seat or pad.

2. Take a few whole breaths, virtually filling the center with air, at that factor actually discharge the breath.

3. Recollect a duration at the same time as you encountered outrage, usually as of overdue. You do not need to pick out your maximum pretty awful scene. Actually, it's insightful initially some element littler. Imagine and experience what passed off, allowing yourself to revel in the outrage once more, at this 2d. Enable the inclination to get as strong as manageable indoors 1 / 4 of protection (e.G., no longer coming to the coronary heart of the trouble in that you want to stand up and shout and hop round!).

4. Different emotions, for instance, problem or dread, might also additionally grow to be you keep in mind the scene. For the existing, check whether or not or no longer or not you may stay with the sentiment outrage.

5. Where on your body do you stumble upon it? Investigate this inclination. You is probably enticed to attempt to push it away. Rather, find out the manner it feels, seeing gross and unpretentious sensations. As you spot a sensation, ask whether or not or now not it increments or declines in pressure. Does it change or pass? Is it warmness or cool?

6. Work on conveying sympathy to the outrage. The sentiment outrage is latest, a few a part of being human. We as an entire ordeal it on occasion. Check whether or not or now not you may assist your very very very own outrage like a mother assisting an little one. What takes place on the off hazard which you hold it thusly, with delicacy and care?

7. Say farewell to the inclination. Gradually take your consideration lower again to the breath and stay with it for some time, giving your emotions a threat to sink into the massive duration of your breath and mindfulness.

8. After you complete, mirror. Which sensations did you notice for your body? Did they alternate as you recall you studied them? Is it proper which you were equipped to deliver sympathy to the outrage? How ought to you try this? What befell to the outrage by the usage of way of then?

Recover from Work Stress in Three Easy Ways

#1: Learn the way to look at your personal passionate reactions.

We can alternate the manner we manage conditions we do now not have manipulate over. "Your authoritative scenario might not be in particular sound, however as an opportunity you may be," Hunter says.

Perceiving and recognizing what you're absolutely managing at artwork is an important preliminary step.

#2: Learn to unwind.

At the factor whilst stretch is hitting you each day, the opportunity of unwinding also can appear to be fantastic. "Yet, putting aside time for yourself is absolutely key," says Hunter. That won't mean you want to take a three-week get-away. Stress assistance is as near inner achieve as a couple of 5-minute stops all through it gradual in which you're tranquil and sensible, honestly being on the time.

#three: Take under consideration that in case you are involved at work, others in your association possibly also are.

That does not advocate decreasing others more slack than you bear in mind yourself, however it technique figuring out a manner to carry down reactivity and lift responsiveness. In distressing airs topics can heighten, but, they do not need to. Any parents can select to be the number one to tone it down.

## Mindful Eating

### 1) Let your body make up for out of vicinity time for your thoughts

Eating short past whole and disregarding your frame's symptoms and symptoms as opposed to backing off and consuming and ceasing whilst your frame says its entire.

Backing off is splendid in evaluation to notable approaches we are capable of get our psyche and frame to supply what we in reality require for nourishment. The body in reality sends its satiation motion around 20 minutes after the thoughts, it's the cause we frequently unknowingly gorge. Be that as it may, on the off threat that we back down, you can permit your body to make up for out of vicinity time on your cerebrum and concentrate the signs and symptoms to eat the nice sum. Basic procedures to backtrack might also very well include take after a huge range of your grandma's behavior, together with taking a seat to consume, biting every chomp 25 instances (or all of the extra), putting your fork down among nibbles, and each this form of antique conduct which is probably likely not as trivial as they seemed. What are some techniques you can back down eating and concentrate all the greater profoundly to your frame's signs and symptoms

2) Know your body's near domestic craving indicators

Is it correct to say which you are reacting to a passionate need or reacting for your body's wishes?

Frequently we concentrate first to our brains, however like severa mindfulness hones, we can also discover extra facts through the usage of tuning into our our bodies first. Instead of really ingesting while we get passionate symptoms, which might be exquisite for each humans, be they stretch, bitterness, dissatisfaction, dejection or perhaps actually weariness, we can song in to our our our bodies. Is your stomach snarling, power low, or feeling actually woozy? Again and once more, we devour at the same time as our mind instructs us to, in preference to our our bodies. Genuine careful consuming is sincerely listening profoundly to our frame's symptoms and symptoms for hunger. Ask your self: What are your frame's yearning alerts, and what are your enthusiastic urge for food triggers?

3) Develop adhering to an incredible healthy dietweight-reduction plan conditions

Eating by myself and arbitrarily instead of Eating with others at set situations and spots

Another way that we devour thoughtlessly is thru way of meandering round searching through cabinets, ingesting indiscriminately instances and places, in location of in truth taking into account our suppers and tidbits. This backs us off for a pleasing some aspect, however maintains us from growing strong natural indicators about what and the quantity to devour, and wires our brains for brand spanking new activates for eating that no longer usually best. (could you definitely want to make a propensity to consume on every occasion you get in the car, or exceptional activities?) Sure, we as a whole chunk from time to time, however it could useful resource each your mind and frame's fitness, additionally alternatively helping your inclination and rest calendar to eat at predictable instances and spots. Truly, this means that taking a seat (at a table!), placing sustenance on a plate or bowl, now not consuming it out of the compartment, and using utensils now not our arms. It likewise eats with others, similarly to the truth which you are sharing and getting some sturdy association, however you furthermore backpedal and can understand the sustenance and dialogue more, and we take our signs and signs from our supper associate, now not finished or undereating out of feeling.

When we positioned our sustenance away in shelves and the cooler, we likewise will likely consume sound measures of robust nourishment, so undergo in thoughts what's around, wherein it is and whether or not or no longer it's far in find out. In the event that we restriction consuming to kitchen and residing room vicinity, we are moreover more averse to devour carelessly or consume whilst multitasking. At the factor even as nourishment is round, we devour it. Furthermore, sustenance, now not typically the maximum satisfactory, is often spherical on the sports.

There are many reasons that the raisin consuming it's miles the sort of succesful exercising, but one is that after we back off and eat sound nourishments like raisins, we often understand them extra than the story we inform ourselves concerning stable sustenances.

You do not want to format your sustenance all the manner right all the way down to each chomp, and its crucial to be adaptable specifically at brilliant activities, but sincerely understand approximately the manner that you could exchange your nutritional patterns at various instances of 365 days or for numerous activities. What's extra, at the same time as you do put together, you are moreover extra prone to consume the sum your frame needs at that point than undereating and reveling later, or indulging and wondering two times about it later.

Exemplary exhortation is to likewise not maintain while hungry, however as an alternative the center way applies proper proper right here too. A highbrow impact known as "moral allowing" has examined that clients who purchase kale will probably then make a beeline for the liquor or frozen yogurt area than the folks who do now not. We count on that our karma will offset and we are able to "spend" it on garbage sustenance, or fantastic not as lots as first-class practices.

four) Eat nourishment no longer memories

Eating nourishments which may be truely ameliorating in place of consuming sustenances which is probably nutritiously stable

This is some unique precarious adjust, and in an brilliant global we will find out feeding sustenances which might be additionally fun and frightening. In any case, preserve in mind that first cautious raisin. Did that appear to be attractive in advance than you attempted it? There are many motives that the raisin ingesting it's miles such an excessive workout, but one is that after we back down and devour robust nourishments like raisins, we often recognize them greater than the story we tell ourselves regarding sound sustenances. As we artwork on eating extra extraordinary and a more noteworthy series sustenances, we're plenty less disposed to orgy on our solace nourishments, and additional slanted to recognize sound nourishments, at final locating numerous nourishments rationally and physical attractive in desire to best a couple.

5) Consider the existence cycle of your sustenance

Considering wherein nourishment originates from rather than thinking about nourishment a finished stop end result.

Unless you are a seeker gatherer or sustenance agriculturist, we've got all have end up out to be commonly detached from our nourishment as of late. A massive type of us don't appreciably reflect onconsideration on in which as a supper originates from beyond the general keep bundling. This is a misfortune, since ingesting gives a mind boggling chance to interface us all the more profoundly to the normal international, the components and to every one-of-a-kind.

When we respite to remember the bulk of the overall population engaged with the supper that has touched base in your plate, from the friends and family (and your self) who set it up, to the individuals who loaded the racks, to the people who planted and collected the crude fixings, to the individuals who bolstered them, it's miles difficult to no longer revel in every thankful and interconnected. Be aware about the water, soil, and specific additives that had been a piece of its advent as you take a seat to consume some thing you are eating. You can hold in mind the social conventions that presented to you this sustenance, the components liberally shared from partners, or added from a miles off vicinity and time to be a exceeded on within the circle of relatives.

As you don't forget everything that went into the dinner, it subsequently finally ends up obviously smooth to involvement and offer manner to the majority of the overall population who gave their danger and exertion, the additives of the universe that contributed their offer, our companions or precursors who shared additives or maybe the creatures who may also furthermore have given their lives to a bit of making this dinner party. With simplest pretty extra mindfulness like this, we can also moreover begin to determine more clever choices approximately manageability and health in our nourishment, no longer nice for us however as an opportunity for the whole planet.

6) Attend in your plate

Occupied ingesting in choice to honestly eating

Multitasking and eating is a components for now not having the capacity to pay attention profoundly to our body's needs and goals. We've all had the experience of avoiding to the movies with our % brimming with popcorn, and in advance than the approaching sights are finished, we're soliciting who ate all from our popcorn. When we are diverted, it finally ends up exceptionally greater tough to music in to our frame's signs and symptoms and signs and signs about nourishment and superb desires. With your next dinner, attempt unmarried-entrusting and really eating, without any displays or diversions apart from getting a fee out of the enterprise you're providing a supper and discussion to.

## Chapter 11: Religious Emotional

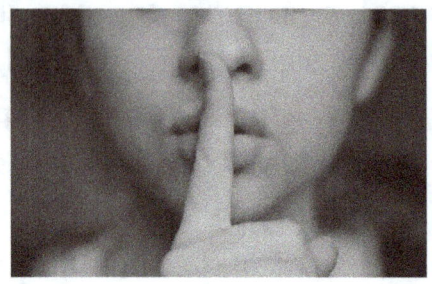

Beliefs, on the facet of fashionable morals, are the principles of who we're and what we stand for. Everyone has a hard and speedy of beliefs that guide their lives, that fuels their passions and tames their internal beasts.

Becoming aware of those beliefs; what they may be, what they recommend to you and the way they have got an effect to your way of lifestyles, is pinnacle in attaining an reputation of your words, for you can't be aware about what you're announcing till you absolutely apprehend what it's far you are announcing.

To try this, reproduction down the following questions and fill in 5 ideals or morals that you have. Consider the textbook meaning of the beliefs (some research may be required). Then, do not forget what they propose to you? Do they suit up? Are they in step with one another?

1. What are your ideals?

2. What is the textbook definition of each perception?

three. What does each belief propose to you?

four. Is this a perception of your or one that you were taught to definitely be given as authentic with?

5. How do you in fact feel approximately this perception?

Lastly, ask your self, "Am I in compliance with my beliefs"? Just because we remember something doesn't make it proper. On that equal be aware, surely because of the fact we're announcing we acquire as authentic with some element, doesn't mean we do. As kids, we are raised to suppose, act and speak a certain way. These teachings grow to be our preliminary beliefs regularly, they are the general beliefs of the society that has been accompanied to keep away from offending every different and despite the fact that we won't simply test them, we take shipping of them to be "how it's miles", for that reason making them a part of our ideals no matter our personal evaluations.

In this 2d, reflect for your list and decide whether or now not the ideals and morals you have got listed are sincerely yours and that you definitely be given as authentic with in them.

Now, undergo in mind the subsequent...

Leo is ready within the customer support line at a large department shop. The clerk in the again of the table is new, this is her first solo shift, and she or he's the only one at the desk; so topics are slow and he or she or he stumbles over the process a chunk. The line is prolonged and Leo has someplace to be in an hour.

Once he eventually gets as a good buy because the desk along collectively together with his move lower back, however, he discovers he does no longer have his receipt. The clerk explains that there is a industrial business enterprise agency insurance that does not allow for the pass again of any devices without a proper receipt, and there is no way for her to generate a few exclusive duplicate.

Leo will become disillusioned, he tells the clerk that she has a terrible gadget and that she is offering terrible customer support due to the truth he doesn't have his receipt and he doesn't believe the commercial enterprise enterprise's policy.

After growing tired of being attentive to the clerk apologize and repeat the insurance, Leo demands to look a supervisor. The clerk calls for the manager. The manager comes and once more offers Leo the same speech as the clerk. He tells the Manager that they're doing a terrible venture and they want to each be fired. In addition to this, he started out to slam his hands at the counter and scream foul words at the personnel, and condemning the business enterprise.

The supervisor, because of the fact that the trouble may terrific hold to enhance asked Leo to depart the store, for he turned into now causing a disruption in the peace. Leo left and vowed in no way to move once more.

Now, taking the above situation, compare it to a time even as you have got been sad with a business agency insurance that stopped you from getting what you desired. Consider the organisation clerk or accomplice who informed you of the insurance. Consider the feelings that ran via your thoughts. What did you say to the clerk? How did they reply? How should you sense if someone spoke to you in that manner? How may you have got have been given replied if it were you? How may you have got spoke back if it were your little one? Was it proper for you to mention what you stated? How might also want to you sense if it became stated to you? How would possibly you feel if you have been within the clerk's feature?

Considering your ideals did you act finally? Or did you act on emotion, had been you privy to the assets you stated and the way they'll have affected the alternative character? Or, have been you speakme from an area of anger. Did you apologize to your movement? Or did you brush it off and keep along with your day? Did you be conscious, or even bear in mind the incorrect in your actions?

When we're aware of our movements, we are aware about our beliefs as a end result, allowing us to better display our phrases further to our actions. The subsequent time you're confronted with a state of affairs wherein your emotions are involved, take a second to mirror for your beliefs and then reply consequently. Putting your beliefs into motion is the first step to turning into conscious of others.

Complete the chart above. Take 10 minutes to mirror on perception and reflect. Do your modern-day movements mimic your ideals? Has there ever been a time you've got got long gone in opposition to them? If you may pass decrease again how might you regulate your moves and manipulate your terms?

2. Be Aware of Your Thoughts

Now that you have noted your ideals, it's time to don't forget your mind. Do Your ideals equate to how you suspect?

A famous social perception is that every one were created identical, as a end result, all need to be treated as such. On that be aware, is it right to pick out out? When you permit your self to expect negatively your beginning doorways for bad movements and if your ideals and morals aren't firmly in vicinity then you may find out your self misplaced thinking how did I get to this point? This isn't me.

Having manage over what you located is crucial whilst staying actual on your beliefs. If your morals are sound, then the phrases you speak need to suggest.

Referring to the earlier situation with Leo and the clerk. Take a 2nd to assume, about the scenario. There is a company policy in area that doesn't allow the clerk to take any returns without a proper receipt. Thus, she can not offer him back his coins. The clerk is an partner; she did now not make up the insurance barring Leo's cross lower back. Her task because of the fact the customer service clerk is to implement the regulations irrespective of how many can also enjoy. So, does she need to be spoken to in an competitive manner?

In this situation, Leo did no longer think about his morals and ideals, therefore he did now not do not forget their emotions of the woman and the supervisor he changed into appealing. Had he have stopped to reflect on his morals be for talking, he might have come to a more rational manner of speaking his thoughts of the store's insurance in a extra humane and rational manner.

By understanding the significance of getting your thoughts replicate your beliefs your phrases will become greater conscious.

Think lower lower back to a time whilst you had bad mind approximately an occasion or a person. Were the ones mind warranted? How can also additionally need to you have had been given grew to end up those horrific thoughts into excellent reinforcement and or reconstructive complaint?

three. Be Aware of Your Feelings

Emotions can also cloud our mind therefore hindering us to recognition on our beliefs due to this taking a long way from us being conscious. When you are aware you're at peace, you do no longer permit traumatic conditions to cloud your judgment and act out of line. Instead, you construct a rational and enlarge a manner to higher react to the scenario being aware of not actually your personal emotions however the emotions of those around you.

When being privy to your emotions, you can higher manipulate the phrases you speak.

If Leo ought to have stopped to anticipate, there may be a danger he could have been greater privy to the situation and taken into attention his phrases. In which he also can have amassed extra data from the clerk and manager approximately his situation and his alternatives on getting delight. Also, he would have spared his picture. When Leo exploded on the clerk and manager, he did now not high-quality disgrace them for now not best being capable of meet his needs, but he shamed himself as not being a rational person, capable of coming to a selection while not having the state of affairs decorate.

By being aware about our emotions, we in addition toughen our ideals and permit ourselves to become extra conscious of the state of affairs. To live within the 2d, one need to release all that motives strain and worry, this shows gaining manage of one's feelings. To do that one want to come to be aware of what they will be. In the example of Leo, he turn out to be disappointed because of the fact he became no longer capable of reap a pass decrease returned.

Think lower lower back to a time at the same time as you allowed your feelings to cloud your beliefs? How did this cast off from your mindfulness? What are you capable of do to save you this inside the destiny?

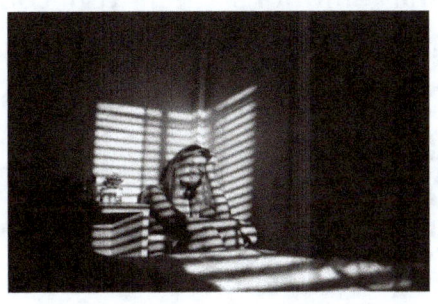

## Chapter 12: Consider Your Actions

1.  Be Aware of What You Do

Actions talk louder than phrases, people will undergo in thoughts you for what your moves greater regularly than for what you say. However, your terms can fuel your movements, like your mind gasoline your emotions. If you permit yourself to grow to be out of touch collectively with your beliefs and your emotions, then you could cloud your recognition of your responses, as a result hindering you from being capable of act in a conscious way.

By being aware of your actions, you may higher manage how you reply to the the ones round you. Being aware of your private movements offers you more private responsibility and permits you to reply rationally to the sector round you.

Analyzing your body language is one manner of pinpointing the way you reply to the the ones around you. When you live in the moment, you discover inner peace. Going thru life disillusioned all of the time ends in a existence of grief. Being aware of what one does can result in a existence of fulfillment and happiness.

Awareness of your physical responses, body language, and frame positioning can allow for the expulsion of negative vibes, this permitting you to live within the second and come to be extra aware and privy to the world around you.

What is the "dumbest" element that you have ever finished? What is the "smartest" factor you have got ever completed? How did they make you sense ultimately? Do you remorse doing each of them? Were you aware of what you've got been doing whilst you have been going it?

2. Be Aware of What You Do to Yourself

The identical way you need to be aware of the way you talk; you want to moreover be aware about what you do. Channeling your ideals, mind, and phrases can offer beneficial resource in guiding your actions.

Taking a deep breath and stepping again from a excessive-stress scenario will will assist you to test the immediate you're in and responding in your emotions will higher prepare you to deal with them. If you allow yourself to be disillusioned you may be dissatisfied, in case you allow your self to be satisfied then you will be happy.

When you are upset do you get angry? Do you yell, scream, cuss; or do you aspect the finger and find reasons why someone else is responsible for the way you sense? By turning into indignant you come to be a ways flung for the prevailing second, consequently allowing yourself to become crushed and pressured. Instead, it is extraordinary to take a step decrease again and examine situations, emerge as aware of what it is you're concerned in and a way to reply to them. Thus, living in the second, acknowledging the area round you and accepting the situation for what it is.

Think over again to a time you made a "idiot" of yourself. How did you feel? How did the ones spherical you reply? Do your movements nonetheless study you? Do human beings however remind you of it? Are you or had been you capable of flow into beyond it?

three.   Be Aware of How You Present Yourself

In is the arena we live in; first impressions are everything. Regardless of methods an lousy lot we faux they'll be now not. If we allow out terrible thoughts, phrases, and actions to govern us, people will recall that we're bad people. The more aware of our surroundings we're, the more we've got control of our movements, for that reason giving us the very last say in who we're and select to be.

When you prevent your self from stressing in a immoderate-stress situation, you allow you present your self as reserved.

When you permit yourself to have a test the glass as 1/2 of complete in vicinity of half of empty, you gift yourself as fantastic.

Becoming aware about who you're, permits you to grow to be aware of the people spherical you and their perception of you. This can also higher your vanity in the long run. Many can also additionally say to no care about what others can also say about you. And that is actual, however, considering one-of-a-type people's belief of you may permit yourself more opportunities in lifestyles. This does not propose permit human beings to outline you.

Becoming aware of the perceptions of those spherical you can will can help you recognition on extra fun elements of existence.

Recall a time even as you acted out of person, or out of what others taken into consideration relevant. How did you revel in in a while? Do you desire you can bypass lower decrease back and change some element, should you? Do you continue to stay on it, regardless of how lengthy within the beyond it changed into? Why do you suspect that is Don't Take Things to Heart

## 1. Be Aware That It Is Easy to Be Wrong

It is straightforward to be incorrect, no person is right. The key's being capable of be given at the same time as you are wrong. Dealing with being wrong does not should be a shot at you as someone. Being wrong does now not outline you, nor does it have an effect on who you're. Not being able to be given on the same time as you're wrong is what starts offevolved to outline you. It's a person flaw that we as people can consequences manipulate, but, we do now not due to the fact it's far much less complicated to get disappointed and make excuses in area of accepting what we lack and addressing it head on.

By acknowledging that you are not great, you allow yourself the liberty of strain and permit yourself to appearance past the faults. Accepting while you're wrong and walking towards answers, permits you to seize the moment and come to be aware about no longer great yourself but of the those spherical you. Providing a diploma of contentment and a revel in of private accomplishment. It suggests that you are the larger character and which you are reserved. The a good buy less stressful conditions you're a part of, the greater you could experience existence and live within the 2nd.

Think about a time on the equal time as you've got been incorrect, who corrected you? How did you reply? Was your response warranted? If given the risk, may you have got spoke back in a selected manner?

## 2. Be Aware That We Need to Be Reminded

When we are corrected, it isn't always due to the fact we're insufficient, it's miles to decorate us as individuals. If you're taking to coronary coronary heart every piece of criticism you get maintain of, you may in no manner expand.

Have you ever been advised that you are operating too sluggish, in spite of the fact which you don't forget that you are working as rapid as humanly possible? Or, have you ever ever ever ever been knowledgeable that your typical average performance is sub par and which you have room for improvement? Have you ever been denied a danger at advancement and been instructed, you aren't the right healthy, or that your skills aren't polished sufficient?

Instead of seeing theses as rejections or jabs at your capabilities, use them as studying opportunities, grow to be privy to your flaws and what you lack. Becoming aware of your weaknesses permits you the possibility to artwork on enhancing them.

Before you get mad at the hiring manager and give you reasons why they omitted you, recall the feedback you have got been given and paintings inside the course of assembly it. Instead of growing with excuses why you are not able to paintings as speedy because of the fact the others broaden some other approach of completing the undertaking without violating protocol.

Remembering that everybody need reminders, that we are not all best, that everybody have flaws, that every person make mistakes, is what lets in us to stay inside the second, seize it for what it's far and turn out to be aware about the matters around us.

## Chapter 13: Don't Jump

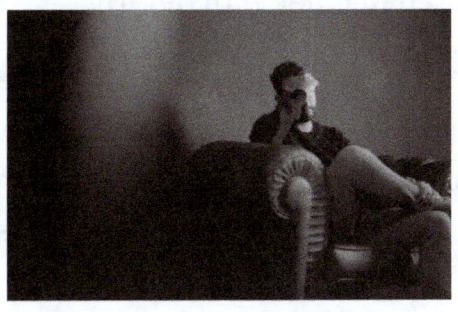

1.  Be Aware of The Miracles that Happen Around You

Miracles take place each day. A toddler is born, an egg hatches, a flower blossoms, and the sector turns. If we attention on every awful issue that comes our way we're able to by no means break out the lure of ache that comes-with-it. However, if we take the time to apprehend existence and stay within the now we are in a function if you want to pinpoint the various miracles that make lifestyles certainly worth living.

It's k which you did no longer get that beautify, notwithstanding your monetary worry you've got managed to make it this a protracted manner with out it.

It's top enough which you had been no longer selected to be the lead singer within the choir, your company despite the fact that went to nationals and your name come to be despite the fact that on the flyer.

It's right sufficient that your courting fell idea, he/she isn't the handiest character in the international you can discover happiness with, you without a doubt need to simply accept that topics show up for a motive and now you have were given a danger to begin glowing.

Being aware that there may be an upside to the entirety will permit you to live inside the 2d, don't stay on what is finished, reside on what's going to be and the way you'll improve to the subsequent step.

Think of 5 miracles that seem each day and why they will be considered miracles, what blessings do they provide to you? How does spotting the ones miracles assist you to live inside the 2d?

2.  Be Aware of The Might in Small Acts

Have you ever come domestic from work exhausted from the day and a loved one has prepared a domestic cooked meal? Have you ever did not understand a idea for college and a person took the time to offer an cause of it until you may recognize? Have you ever lengthy past to a coffee store and the individual earlier than you paid in your drink earlier than you even got to the sign in?

These small acts of kindness ought to make or destroy each person's day. Taking the time to just be satisfactory to someone and help better their modern-day situation, no matter how small the project is will, in the long run, have an first rate have an impact on on on the character, and an excellent higher influence on you.

By being aware about the small subjects you could do to decorate someone's day you permit your self to percent the thrill of residing within the 2nd and being privy to others. By committing small acts of kindness, you display that you are compassionate and therefore aware and aware about the emotions of others. I task you to do some aspect tremendous for a loved one or possibly a stranger. It doesn't want to be something huge, only a easy gesture to expose which you care. You might probably wash the dishes, easy a room, prepare dinner a meal, or perhaps purchase a person a espresso. The alternatives are countless; you just want to do it from the coronary heart without looking ahead to something else in cross returned; then will you be living in the second.

Think of strategies you may stay inside the 2nd at the same time as developing a small gesture to enhance someone else's day.

Make a listing of five small subjects that you can do, who you could do it for and the way it is able to brighten their day.

Chapter four we're aware about what we take delivery of as real with and we recognize how our emotions have an impact on our actions, thoughts, and terms we're greater capable of taking manipulate of them and redirecting the negatives into positives. If no individual else, we are liable for ourselves.

When there is a midterm due, it is as a good buy as us to finish it.

When faced with war, it is as lots as us on how we reply.

When we are wrong it's far as a whole lot as us to really accept it and try and correct it.

The greater responsible we're for ourselves, the more capable we are of playing brilliant inside the moment for what it's far and now not living at the awful.

Consider a time while you had the danger to be responsible for your movements. Where you? How did you respond? If you weren't how what need to you have got were given finished in any other case?

## 2.Be Aware of Who You Are Becoming

Another element of becoming greater conscious and aware of the prevailing 2d is to be privy to who you're. What makes you glad? What are your triggers? What are your fears? The extra you are in music with yourself, the higher you can carry out your beliefs, the better you may take shipping of your flaws, and the better you could artwork within the direction of evolving.

Becoming aware about who you are is essential in phrases of growing yourself right right into a conscious being. At the stop of the day, if you may't change everybody else if you can't help every person else. You can simplest help yourself, you could only change yourself.

## Chapter 14: Making The Most Of Now!

"The only way to survive eternity is to be able to appreciate each moment."

Lauren Kate, Fallen

When we prepare ourselves to live in every minute, we submerge ourselves in it and start to find its magnificence and marvel. We learn center and how to deal with our vitality. Proficient competitors comprehend and utilize this sort of concentrate extremely well. They realize that achievement and achievement are an aftereffect of the handy administration and adjusting of vitality.

To make the most of each minute we should grasp it. All that we do and each individual we interact with merits our full consideration. Notwithstanding while resting we ought to enjoy the experience. It gives us the chance to energize, restore and pick up clarity.

Regularly we put colossal desires on ourselves and our lives. We race to do this, hustle just a bit with that, without really getting a charge out of the procedure. What's the hurry? Where do we believe we're going? On the off chance that we don't stop and consider where we're at, we're presumably overlooking what's really important. Rather, when we welcome every minute and accumulate the lessons from it, we live intentionally, deliberately and dependably.

Obviously, this doesn't mean we don't have to arrange, set objectives or get ready for what's to come. We can do these things and still appreciate every minute as it unfurls.

For example, in the event that we have set an objective to practice every day, we would continue with it while getting a charge out of the genuine procedure, or minute, of working out (or if nothing else be at the time of it).

In like manner, when we live in the past and don't relinquish agonizing encounters, saw wrongs, or troublesome times, we sentence ourselves to a present and eventual fate of the same. We can't change the past. We can, nonetheless, grapple with it, realize that it's over, and proceed onward.

Living at the time implies relinquishing the past and confiding later on. When we are sure and idealistic in the present, we open the likelihood of a positive and promising future. We deserve to make the most of each minute - now!

Benefits You Receive When You Live for the Moment

• You turn out to be more associated with your musings and sentiments

• Are more associated with others

• Feel more appreciation and happiness regarding life

•On the off chance that you live at the time, it won't cruise you by

•Feel more engaged, quiet and alive

•Feel less on edge and dreadful

Techniques for Living for the Moment

•Train your psyche to concentrate on the present movement.

•Take part in, and feel what you are doing. Appreciate the procedure.

•Learn unwinding procedures keeping in mind the end goal to be available in every minute.

•Pay heed to your surroundings - sights, sounds, smells, mood.

•Listen mindfully to the discussion of others, music, even quiet.

•Relish your sustenance and beverage. Taste every piece.

Like all aptitudes, preparing yourself to appreciate and live at the time requires some serious energy and practice. Start now and see life from a new, new point of view.

## Chapter 15: Practicing Mindfulness

"Do not dwell in the past, do not dream of the future, concentrate the mind on the present moment. "

Buddha

Being mindful of the present moment was initially created in the Buddhist conventions of Asia, however today is utilized as a system as a part of which a man turns out to be deliberately and non-judgmentally mindful of their contemplations and activities right now.

It is the act of monitoring ourselves without becoming involved with pondering the past or agonizing over what's to come. One of the enormous difficulties we confront in this quick paced, always showing signs of change world is to be available in our own particular lives. We have a tendency to get so made up for lost time in the free for all of what's happening around us that we regularly neglect what's going on at the time.

Why would that be an issue? It's an issue in light of the fact that on an everyday premise it causes us anxiety, wear and tear and gets to be negative to our physical and enthusiastic wellbeing.

In like manner, left unchecked the brain can meander and unleash a wide range of negative musings and feelings including outrage, desires, envy, wretchedness and endless others. Be that as it may, working on being careful can outfit and deal with those considerations and advance mindfulness and internal quiet.

Scientists who have considered the impacts of the individuals who hone care found that the subjects for the most part experience less negative feelings, are more upbeat and idealistic, and have all the more even left-right mind movement.

1.Begin by trying. Roll out a guarantee to improvement the propensities for surging, working indiscriminately and not focusing.

Notice regions where you are not being careful.

2.Moderate down. Take a full breath before starting an action, regardless of what it is, and concentrate on the procedure.

3.Watch yourself. On the off chance that the present minute includes stress, watch your considerations and feelings and how they influence your body. Notice when your contemplations are diverting you from the present minute.

4.Practice. Get work on being careful by performing an undertaking you as a rule do eagerly or unknowingly, for example, brushing your teeth, and do it carefully.

Being careful doesn't mean you'll never be in a rush, have irritating considerations and feelings, or not have the capacity to accomplish more than one thing without a moment's delay. It only implies that you'll be doing all of them all the more deliberately.

You will have more knowledge and consciousness of your decisions and your capacity to improve ones will be upgraded. To have a more settled, more agreeable presence, make the dedication today to be more careful and mindful of all that you do.

Your thoughts are not always you

Life unfurls in the present. In any case, so frequently, we let the present disappear, permitting time to surge past surreptitiously and unseized, and wasting the valuable seconds of our lives as we stress over the future and ruminate about what's past. Buddhist researcher B. Alan Wallace says, "We're living in a world that contributes significantly to mental discontinuity, crumbling, diversion, decoherence". We're continually accomplishing something, and we permit little time to practice stillness and quiet.

When we're grinding away, we fantasize about being on furlough; in the midst of a furlough, we stress over the work heaping up on our work areas. We harp on meddling recollections of the past or fuss about what might happen later on. We don't value the living present in light of the fact that our "monkey minds," as Buddhists call them, vault from thought to thought like monkeys swinging from tree to tree.

The vast majority of us don't attempt our considerations in mindfulness. Or maybe, our considerations control us. Keeping in mind the end goal to feel more in control of our brains and our lives, to discover the feeling of parity that evades us, we have to venture out of this current, to delay, and to rest in stillness—to quit doing and concentrate on simply being.

We have to live more at the time. Living at the time—additionally called care—is a condition of dynamic, open, deliberate consideration on the present. When you get to be careful, you understand that you are not your musings; you turn into an onlooker of your considerations from minute to minute without passing judgment on them. Being mindful about the moment you are in includes neither being with your contemplations as they seem to be, neither getting a handle on at them nor pushing them away. Rather than releasing your life by without living it, you stir to encounter.

Developing a nonjudgmental consciousness of the present gives a large group of advantages. Care diminishes stress, supports insusceptible working, lessens incessant agony, brings down circulatory strain, and helps patients adapt to growth. By lightening stress, spending a couple of minutes a day effectively concentrating on living at the time decreases the danger of coronary illness.

Careful individuals are more satisfied, more overflowing, more compassionate, and more secure. They have higher self-regard and are all the more tolerating of their own shortcomings. Securing mindfulness in the without a moment's hesitation diminishes the sorts of impulsivity and reactivity that underlie sadness, voraciously consuming food, and consideration issues. Careful individuals can hear negative criticism without feeling debilitated. They battle less with their sentimental accomplices and are all the more obliging and less guarded. Therefore, careful couples have all the more fulfilling connections.

Living at the time includes a significant conundrum: You can't seek after it for its advantages. That is on account of the desire of prize dispatches a future-arranged attitude, which subverts the whole procedure. Rather, you simply need to trust that the prizes will come. There are numerous ways to care—and at the center of each is a Catch 22. Humorously, relinquishing what you need is the best way to get it.

## Chapter 16: How To Live Stress-Free And In The Moment

"If there's one thing I learned, it's that nobody is here forever. You have to live for the moment, each and every day . . . the here, the now."

Simone Elkeles, Perfect Chemistry

While I have shared with you all that you are required to know about being in the moment, in this chapter, I help you understand how you can live stress free when you are living in the moment. The tips shared in this chapter can only help you achieve what you are after if you practice them on a daily basis and not have breaks in between. Once you get the hang of it, these tips will automatically become an essential part of your life and your daily routine.

1.Begin little by little. While you may be enticed to totally redesign your way of life, it is not important to roll out huge improvements to begin living at the time. Begin by consolidating new propensities each one in turn. When you have a feeling that you have aced a propensity, include something else.

2.For instance, rather than attempting to contemplate for 20 minutes for each day immediately, begin by attempting to ruminate for three minutes for each day. At that point, expand your time as you turn out to be more OK with reflection. Stroll to work with your telephone in your pocket. Don't content or chat on the telephone unless it is a crisis.

3.Divert your brain when it meanders. It is typical for your brain to meander, yet with a specific end goal to live at the time, you have to keep your psyche concentrated on the present. When you see that your brain is meandering, use tender redirection to concentrate on the present once more.

Recognize that your psyche is meandering without judging yourself for doing as such.

4. Try not to get angry with yourself if your brain meanders. It is ordinary for your psyche to meander here and there. Simply acknowledge that you took somewhat mental excursion and return your center to the present.

5. Pick a care signal. It might be hard to recollect to be careful when you are exceptionally occupied. A care prompt, for example, a string that is tied around your wrist, or a coin in your shoe a pen mark on your hand, can help you to recall to be careful. When you see the signal, ensure that you pause for a minute to stop and notice your environment. You can likewise utilize something more outside like making some tea, looking in the mirror, or evacuating your shoes after work as your sign. Before long, you may start to disregard the sign since you are utilized to it. In the

event that this happens, change your signal to something else.

6.Grin and chuckle all the more frequently. Living at the time can be a test on the off chance that you are in a terrible state of mind or simply feeling somewhat down, however grinning and chuckling can improve you feel even you compel yourself to grin and laugh. If you find that you are not centered around the present since you feel troubled, constrain yourself to grin and giggle a bit. Regardless of the fact that you put on a fake grin and giggle foolishly, you ought to begin to feel better immediately.

7.Do kind things for others. Performing irregular demonstrations of benevolence can help you to live at the time by refocusing your consideration on what's going on before you. Search for little things that you can do to show consideration to others. The kind demonstrations that you perform will help you to back off and see your environment.

8.For instance, you could offer a compliment to an outsider. Look for approaches to show consideration in whatever circumstance you are in. Notwithstanding something as straightforward as grinning and gesturing at individuals for the duration of the day may light up somebody's day and keep you concentrated on the present.

9.Do one thing at once. Single-assignment, don't multi-undertaking. When you're pouring water, simply pour water. When you're eating, simply eat. When you're washing, simply bathe. Try not to attempt to knock off a couple assignments while eating or washing or driving. A famous Zen adage: "When walking, walk. Whenever eating, eat."

10.Concentrate on what is currently, quit stressing over what's to come. Turned out to be more mindful of your reasoning - would you say you are continually stressing over what's to come? Figure out how to perceive when you're doing this, and after that work on taking yourself back to the present. Simply concentrate on what you're doing, at this moment. Appreciate the present minute.

11.In the event that something is irritating you, move toward it instead of far from it (acknowledgment). We as a whole have torment in our lives, whether it's the ex despite everything we yearn for, the jackhammer growling over the road, or the sudden flood of uneasiness when we get up to give a discourse. On the off chance that we let them, such aggravations can divert us from the happiness regarding life. Incomprehensibly, the undeniable reaction—concentrating on the issue keeping in mind the end goal to battle and overcome it—frequently aggravates it.

12.To capitalize on time, forget about it (flow).Perhaps the most finish method for living at the time is the condition of aggregate ingestion therapists call stream.

164

Stream happens when you're so immersed in an errand that you forget about everything else around you. Stream exemplifies an evident Catch 22: How would you be able to live at the time in case you not in any case mindful exist apart from everything else? The profundity of engagement assimilates you intensely, keeping consideration so engaged that diversions can't infiltrate. You concentrate so seriously on what you're doing that you're uninformed of the progression of time. Hours can go without you taking note.

13.Stream is a slippery state. Similarly as with sentiment or rest, you can't simply will yourself into it—everything you can do is set the stage, making the ideal conditions for it to happen.

14.To enhance your execution, quit contemplating it (unselfconsciousness). I've never felt agreeable on a move floor. My developments feel cumbersome. I feel like individuals are passing judgment on me. I never recognize what to do with my arms. I need to give up, yet I can't, on the grounds that I know I look ludicrous. That is the primary mystery of living at the time: Thinking too hard about what you're doing really aggravates you do. In case you're in a circumstance that makes you restless— giving a discourse, acquainting yourself with a more interesting, moving—concentrating on your nervousness has a tendency to increase it.

15.Make cleaning and cooking your contemplation. Cooking and cleaning are regularly seen as drudgery, in any case they are both extraordinary approaches to practice care, and can be incredible customs performed every day. In the event that cooking and cleaning appear like exhausting errands to you, take a stab at doing them as a type of contemplation. Put your whole personality into those assignments, focus, and do them gradually and totally. It could change your whole day (and in addition go out). Continue rehearsing. When you get disappointed, simply take a full breath.

16.When you are conversing with somebody, be available, rationally and physically. What number of us have invested energy with somebody however have been supposing about what we have to do later on? Then again considering what we need to say next, rather than truly listening to that individual? Rather, concentrate on being available, on truly tuning in, on truly making the most of your time with that individual.

17.Spend no less than 5 minutes every day doing nothing. Simply sit peacefully. Gotten to be mindful of your considerations. Concentrate on your relaxing. Notice your general surroundings. Gotten to be OK with the quiet and stillness. It'll do you a ton of good - and just takes 5 minutes!

18.Put space between things. It's a method for dealing with your timetable so that you generally have room schedule-wise to finish every errand. Try not to timetable things near one another - rather, leave room between things on your calendar. That gives you a more casual calendar, and leaves space on the off chance that one errand takes longer than you arranged.

19.Eat gradually and enjoy your food. Food can be packed down our throats in a surge, however where's the delight in that? Enjoy every nibble, gradually, and truly get the most out of your sustenance. Strikingly, you'll eat less thusly, and condensation your sustenance better too.

20.Live gradually and flavor your life. Just as you would relish your nourishment by eating it all the more gradually, do all that along these lines - moderate down and appreciate every single minute. Tune into the sights and sounds and stir your faculties to your general surroundings.

If you practice these above tips on a daily basis, you are sure to notice a drastic improvement in your temperament. You will feel more alive and happy. You will also find yourself with renewed energy to do all the things you want to.

## Chapter 17: Anxiety-Kicking Journey

'Life became by no means imagined to be a struggle.'

Stuart Wilde.

'Nothing within the worldwide is in truth genuinely well worth having or honestly well worth doing besides it way

strive, ache, and trouble.'

Theodore Roosevelt.

WHICH SAYING DO YOU choose? I vote for Stuart Wilde's. If you opted for Roosevelt's this book won't be your cup of tea or flagon of hemlock.

From as younger as seven, I suspected lifestyles must be a laugh, not conflict and strife. Well-meaning humans attempted to persuade me in any other case; life is difficult. Parents, aunts, and Uncle Tom Cobley threw countless clichés at me, which include 'coins no longer developing on timber', and achievement and happiness due to masses of tough art work.

We are more than midway to abundance, fitness and happiness on the same time as we do what makes our souls sing and study intuition. If something feels proper, it generally is. If some element feels incorrect, then ditto.

Outside opinion drowns internal knowingness (instinct). As the announcing is going, you shouldn't pressure a rectangular peg right right into a spherical hole. A film that shows the misery and risk of this is The Dead Poets Society. When we follow our bliss, life is more comfortable. Do what we hate at our peril. Intuition is a green web page visitors mild, announcing flow in advance and a knot in the tummy is a red caution moderate.

I understand, much less complicated stated than finished. I actually have ignored many warning lights and allow extraordinary human beings's common experience speak me out of situations and thoughts that felt right. Every time I allowed this to stand up it added approximately prolonged difficult roads to tour, and hard to transport lower back home from; and I propose 'home' in each a figurative and real revel in.

I'm now not suggesting that if we watch Netflix for hours every day, without doing a scrap to earn a crust, that riches and the correct lifestyles magically appear. However, there are a few subjects we can do, or not do, that make lifestyles greater magical – and much less complicated.

When we are real to ourselves and take note of our internal voice, lifestyles is greater thrilling and abundant. Stuff we enjoy doing does now not seem like difficult paintings. We are greater snug, less forced and happier while we pay attention to our intuition and comply with our hearts.

Much youngsters magic abandoned me as I listened to the well-that means recommendation of pals and loved ones who attempted to manipulate lifestyles from the outside, in preference to following their hearts.

From feeling secure, I sincerely have turn out to be demanding and took on the priority of those round me. Often, human beings count on fear will disappear as quickly as imagined situations are first-rate...

'Life might be ideal if I come to be rich.'

They win the lottery and fear about losing all of it.

'Life is probably fantastic as soon as I skip my examination.'

They get an 'A' and worry approximately failing the subsequent one.

'If I get domestic in a unmarried piece nowadays, I'll never worry approximately driving once more.'

They worry about the subsequent experience as quickly as they park the auto.

We need to get to the deliver of problems; otherwise, it's like having a thirsty plant and watering the leaves now not the basis. Problems are not solved at the extent of the trouble.

Worry is often a symptom of deep-seated strain.

If you've felt sick with tension, the manner annoying it is while a person says, 'Pull yourself together.'

Slap!

An worrying patron stated, 'I choice I had a broken leg or maximum cancers because I'd get empathy from friends and loved ones.'

One of the worst matters about tension is stressful the fear will sound daft to others.

Anxiety is regularly approximately minor topics blown out of percentage: This regularly takes vicinity whilst we bury actual problems or are not right to ourselves. If we don't renowned discontent and do something about it, anxiety bites us on the nostril.

 'The misfortunes toughest to go through are

the ones which by no means came.'

James Russell Lowell.

IN CHURCH, MARRYING my first husband, I knew he became incorrect for me. I come to be only nineteen, but I desired the fairytale I'd projected onto the destiny. His accurate seems lured me, and I imagined residing luckily ever after in a romantic Garden of Eden.

The fact emerge as an lousy lot a whole lot much less than rosy. Instead of a life entire of passion and romance, I lived with a fussy controlling vintage man hidden in a good-looking younger man's frame. The longer I stayed within the marriage, the extra I worried over stuff that sounded ridiculous even to myself.

My GP (General Practitioner) sent me for group remedy. I changed into twenty-three and met a myriad of characters that ranged from careworn to suicidal.

A tearful lady said, 'I can't cope in the kitchen.'

Hello, calling 1952.

## Chapter 18: 'What Can't You Deal With?'

'I can't cope, I can't cope.'

A sixteen-yr-vintage boy emerge as a harm after cramming for assessments. 'It's the use of me loopy.'

'It may strength all and sundry loopy,' I said, remembering 'O' degrees.

'No, this is horrible. I can't even take a look at anymore. The terms come at me.'

'What about a unique, in preference to revision?'

'I can't have a look at one phrase due to the reality I experience infinite associations and my head explodes.'

'How do you suggest?'

'I examine car then have to discover at the same time as the number one vehicle end up made, how the engine labored, what number of makes of motors there are and so forth. That's one phrase then there may be the subsequent and the subsequent. I can't stand it.'

Poor lad.

'Why are you proper here?' I requested a hand-wringing female.

'I maintain imagining horrible things will seem.'

'What type of factors?'

'Accidents, way into the future. I can't experience myself now as there are lousy matters in advance.'

It transpired her husband controlled nearly every element of her lifestyles and he or she involved she'd lose the final of her energy.

'Love every extraordinary, but make not a bond of love: Let it as an opportunity be a moving sea between the beaches of your souls.'

Khalil Gibran, The Prophet.

WOULD THE WORST OF my anxiety go if I left my husband? My former zest for existence grow to be behind bars. If I left the marital jail, the mental prison would possibly fall away. My GP had hinted at this, and I'd left out him, nonetheless clutching to my romantic dream. My medical doctor become clever even as he despatched me to the enterprise wherein there have been human beings with deeper intellectual issues than mine.

My unconscious goaded me to very very personal as tons as the reality, hitting me with larger and huge anxiety sticks. If we don't take note of a message from the universe, it by no means fails to remind us. Thanks!

My marriage limped along for a while after the organization remedy, but I changed into a shadow of my former satisfied self.

Out of the blue, even as we were watching Nanny with Wendy Craig, my husband said, 'I've met a person and need a divorce.'

Before we married, my destiny mum-in-regulation had warned, 'My son's a extremely good lad, however he'll drag you down, break your spirit.'

She meant like herself. She obeyed her husband's each command, squashing her joie de vivre to residence his miserable nature, which modified into, sarcastically, due to anxiety. If his existence wasn't run like a navy regime, he panicked, and actually anybody else needed to fall in together with his orders.

At first, I actually have emerge as disenchanted approximately the upcoming divorce, and my ego come to be a tad harm.

But  days after we break up up I drove to paintings in my blue Ford Fiesta. The sun came out, and Johnny Nash warbled from the radio, 'I can See Clearly Now the Rain

Has Gone.' I had a head-to-toe warmth whoosh of pleasure.

I emerge as more youthful.

I modified into unfastened.

I become happy.

I ought to see certainly now the husband had lengthy lengthy past.

AFTER THAT, THERE WAS one difficulty wherein I had the entirety fabric I should ever need – a wealthy, adorable, second husband and a lavish domestic in primary London.

However, quick the anxieties started out over again: What if this? What if that? Horrific future conditions accomplished in an endless, torturous loop in my head. The horrid sample had repeated.

Does this propose that marriage typically reasons tension? Of course no longer. But not being true to ourselves does. Doing all the compromising does. Not recognition up for ourselves does – now not always over each little detail but in reality essential stuff. Saying sure even as you suggest no, time and again, is the short song to anxiety.

'To be your self in a worldwide this is continuously seeking to make you a few thing else is the great accomplishment.'

Ralph Waldo Emerson.

IF WE DON'T DO WHAT makes our souls sing and always kowtow to one of a kind people's desires, we lose our zest for life. If we live a person else's lifestyles in choice to following our satisfaction, we regularly interest on unrelated anxieties to detract from the actual problems.

When we take a look at our instinct, there may be a snug region inside, like coming home to a warmth house after a tough trek thru the snow in wet clothes and leaky shoes.

No rely how erratic the out of doors worldwide is, there may be protection deep inner. Little children understand this, it's all part of the magic of greater younger youngsters. But at the same time as an excessive amount of out of doors records annoying situations and contradicts our internal knowingness, the experience of inner calm and safety disappears, and panic and fear take over.

My mum lived in an almost everlasting kingdom of excessive-anxiety over trivialities, and I even have become a worried little one.

I can't write High Anxiety without considering the outstanding Mel Brooks movie. Such a cope with. It's set within the 'Psychoneurotic Institute for the Very, Very Nervous' – and might be very, very funny. Check it out if you need a first rate giggle.

Living thru imagined and projected troubles may be worse than any actual occasion.

'We go through extra in imagination than in reality.'

Seneca.

AS A CHILD, I BELIEVED ritual need to stop horrible subjects happening. This is a symptom of OCD (obsessive-compulsive ailment) it honestly is commonplace for worriers. If I didn't touch the door three times in advance than I have been given into mattress a few element terrible might happen. The imaginary horrors numerous. What fun!

Despite those niggles, I turn out to be, within the critical, a sunny infant, however from the age of approximately 9, underlying tension chipped away at my joy.

www.ingramcontent.com/pod-product-compliance
Lightning Source LLC
Chambersburg PA
CBHW071336120626
46546CB00002B/584